Complete Emergency Care

American Safety & Health Institute
With
Human Kinetics

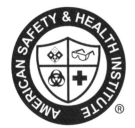

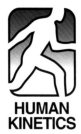

HUMAN
KINETICS

The American Safety & Health Institute
logo is a registered trademark of the
American Safety & Health Institute.

Library of Congress Cataloging-in-Publication Data

Complete Emergency care / American Safety & Health Institute with Human
  Kinetics.
    p. ; cm.
  Includes bibliographical references and index.
  ISBN-13: 978-0-7360-6717-1 (soft cover)
  ISBN-10: 0-7360-6717-5 (soft cover)
  1. Medical emergencies. 2. First aid in illness and injury.
  I. American Safety & Health Institute (Organization). II. Human Kinetics (Organization)
  [DNLM: 1. Emergency Treatment--methods.   WA 292 E515 2007]
  RC86.7.E542 2007
  616.02'5--dc22

ISBN-10: 0-7360-6717-5
ISBN-13: 978-0-7360-6717-1

The Web addresses cited in this text were current as of October 2006, unless otherwise noted.

Managing Editor: Anne Cole
Assistant Editor: Laura Koritz
Copyeditor: Jan Feeney
Proofreader: Julie Marx Goodreau
Indexer: Betty Frizzéll
Permission Manager: Dalene Reeder
Graphic Designer: Nancy Rasmus
Photo Manager: Laura Fitch
Cover Designer: Keith Blomberg
Photographer (cover): Neil Bernstein
Photographer (interior): Figure 2.9 Custom Medical Stock Photo: figures 5.1-5.7, 5.11-5.12, and photo on page 152 by Jill White; all others provided by American Safety & Health Institute
Art Manager: Kelly Hendren
Illustrator: Figure 5.9 by Kelly Hendren; figure 5.10 by Al Wiborn; all others provided by American Safety & Health Institute
Printer: United Graphics

Printed in the United States of America   10   9   8   7   6   5   4   3   2

Human Kinetics
Web site: www.HumanKinetics.com

United States: Human Kinetics, P.O. Box 5076, Champaign, IL 61825-5076
800-747-4457
e-mail: humank@hkusa.com

Canada: Human Kinetics, 475 Devonshire Road, Unit 100, Windsor, ON N8Y 2L5
800-465-7301 (in Canada only)
e-mail: orders@hkcanada.com

Europe: Human Kinetics, 107 Bradford Road, Stanningley
Leeds LS28 6AT, United Kingdom
+44 (0) 113 255 5665
e-mail: hk@hkeurope.com

Australia: Human Kinetics, 57A Price Avenue, Lower Mitcham, South Australia 5062
08 8372 0999
e-mail: info@hkaustralia.com

New Zealand: Human Kinetics, Division of Sports Distributors NZ Ltd.
P.O. Box 300 226 Albany, North Shore City, Auckland
0064 9 448 1207
e-mail: info@humankinetics.co.nz

contents

preface

chapter 1   Bloodborne Pathogens

The American Safety & Health Institute (ASHI) is an association of professional safety and health educators providing nationally recognized training programs across the United States and in several foreign countries. ASHI's mission is to continually improve safety and health education by promoting high standards for members, principles of sound research for curriculum development, and the professional development of safety and health instructors worldwide.

Standards. This student handbook is based upon the requirements of the U.S. Department of Labor, Occupational Safety & Health Administration Regulations (Standards - 29 CFR). Subpart: Z, Subpart Title: Toxic and Hazardous Substances, Standard Number: 1910.1030 Standard Title: Bloodborne Pathogens. Compliance with this standard requires trainees to have direct access to a qualified trainer during training. The trainer must supplement the training with required site-specific information including the location of the exposure control plan and the procedures to be followed if an exposure incident occurs. Training employees solely by means of providing this handbook, showing a video, or completing a generic computer program without the opportunity for a discussion period is a violation of the standard.[1]

Infection Control Terminology. OSHA 1910.1030 defines the term "universal precautions" as an approach to infection control to treat all human blood and certain human body fluids as if they were known to be infectious for HIV, HBV, and other bloodborne pathogens. In 1996, the U.S. Department of Health and Human Services (HHS) and Centers for Disease Control (CDC) published *Guidelines for Isolation Precautions in Hospitals.*[2] This guideline recommends the use of "standard precautions" to reduce the risk of transmission of bloodborne and other pathogens for the care of all patients in hospitals. Standard precautions combines universal precautions and body substance isolations into a single set of precautions to be used for the care of all patients in hospitals, regardless of their presumed infection status. Isolation practices in U.S. hospitals continue to evolve. In this program, ASHI uses the term universal precautions based on the OSHA Standard. For compliance with OSHA Standards, the use of either universal precautions or standard precautions is acceptable.[3]

Airborne Pathogens. OSHA revoked a proposed standard on Occupational Exposure to Tuberculosis in 2003.[4] Respiratory protection from tuberculosis and other occupational diseases caused by breathing contaminated air requires the establishment of a respiratory protection program and the training of employees in the respiratory hazards to which they are potentially exposed. See OSHA Standard 1910.134 for compliance requirements.

ASHI has used reasonable effort to provide up-to-date, accurate information that conforms to generally accepted recommendations at the time of publication. Science and technology are constantly creating new knowledge and practice. Like any printed material, this publication may become out of date over time. Guidelines for safety and prevention cannot be given that will apply in all cases as the circumstances of each incident often vary widely. *These recommendations supersede recommendations made in previous ASHI programs.* ASHI offers training and certification programs in emergency care and occupational safety and health for corporate America, government agencies, and emergency responders. To learn more about ASHI, visit www.ashinstitute.org.

Municipal, state, provincial, national, or federal regulations are governmental orders having the force of law. In the United States, Canada, and most other industrialized countries, workplace safety regulations and occupational licensing requirements prescribe scope of practice, rules, standards, and conditions that every training agency, program, instructor, and licensed person must comply with. ASHI training centers and their authorized instructors must be completely familiar with the regulations and licensing requirements of persons to whom they offer training and certification. Training Centers and authorized Instructors must not advertise, represent, or otherwise promote that their programs will meet specific regulations or licensing requirements unless and until such is confirmed with the licensing authority and/or ASHI.

References

1. Occupational Safety & Health Administration. Compliance Directive CPL 02-02-069 - CPL 2-2.69 - Enforcement Procedures for the Occupational Exposure to Bloodborne Pathogens 11/27/2001. Available: www.osha.gov/[22 May 2006]

2. Guideline for Isolation Precautions in Hospitals Julia S. Garner, RN, MN, and the Hospital Infection Control Practices Advisory Committee. From the Public Health Service, US Department of Health and Human Services, Centers for Disease Control and Prevention, Atlanta, Georgia. Garner JS, Hospital Infection Control Practices Advisory Commitee. Guideline for isolation precautions in hospitals. *Infect Control Hosp Epidemiol* 1996; 17:53-80, and *Am J Infect Control* 1996; 24:24-52. Available: www.cdc.gov/ncidod/dhqp/gl_isolation_ptI.html [25-Mar-06]

3. Occupational Safety & Health Administration. Hospital eTool - HealthCare Wide Hazards Module, (Lack of) Universal Precautions. Available: www.osha.gov/SLTC/etools/hospital/hazards/univprec/univ.html [25-Mar-06]

4. Occupational Exposure to Tuberculosis; Proposed Rule; Termination of Rulemaking Respiratory Protection for M. Tuberculosis; Final Rule; Revocation - 68:75767-75775 12/31/2003 Available: www.osha.gov/pls/oshaweb/owadisp.show_document?p_table=FEDERAL_REGISTER&p_id=18050 [22-May-06]

chapter 2   Basic First Aid

ASHI is a member of the National First Aid Science Advisory Board cofounded by the American Red Cross and American Heart Association®, Inc., and a contributor to the 2005 Consensus of First Aid Science and Recommendations.

This program contains evidence-based first aid recommendations. "Evidence-based" means recommendations collectively agreed upon by members of the National First Aid Science Advisory Board (NFASAB) to be safe, practical, and effective after a thorough evaluation of the medical science and recommendations based on medical literature. First aid recommendations that reflect NFASAB consensus on peer-reviewed scientific studies are indicated with the letters "COS" for "Consensus on Science." Other evidence-based recommendations and source authorities are referenced by endnote.

The Basic First Aid program is based upon the following standards, guidelines, regulations, protocols, and recommendations:

- ASTM International Standard F 2171-02 *"Standard Guideline Defining the Performance of First Aid Providers in Occupational Settings"* April 2002.

- *Caring for Our Children. National Health and Safety Performance Standards: Guidelines for Out-of-Home Child Care Programs.* 2nd Ed. Copyright 2002 by American Academy of Pediatrics, American Public Health Association, National Resource Center for Health and Safety in Child Care Available: nrc.uchsc.edu/CFOC/XMLVersion/NewTOCwoSubs.xml [3-Mar-05].

- Department of Human Resources and Skills Development (HRSD), Canada Occupational Health and Safety Regulations Part 16 - First Aid Available: www.hrsdc.gc.ca/en/lp/lo/fll/part2/cohsregs/part16.shtml [22-Jul-05].

- *EMSC Partnership for Children/National Association of EMS Physicians Model Pediatric Protocols:* 2003 Revision Pediatrics Committee, National Association of EMS Physicians. *Prehospital Emergency Care* Oct/Dec 2004 Vol. 8, No 4. pgs 343-365.

- *First Aid.* National First Aid Science Advisory Board. 2005 First Aid Science Advisory Board Evidence Evaluation Conference

© 2005 American Heart Association and the American National Red Cross. Circulation. 2005; 112: III-115-III-125.

- *First Aid.* Headquarters, Departments of The Army, The Navy, and The Air Force and Commandant, Marine Corps, Washington, DC, 15 July 2004.

- Guidelines for Cardiopulmonary Resuscitation and Emergency Cardiovascular Care. *Circulation.* 2005; 112:IV-1–IV-211© 2005 American Heart Association®, Inc.

- *First Aid, First On the Scene. The Complete Guide to First Aid and CPR.* 3rd Ed. St. John Ambulance ©2001 Priory of Canada of the Most Venerable Order of the Hospital of St. John of Jerusalem. www.sja.ca.

- U.S. Department of Homeland Security, United States Coast Guard. www.uscg. mil/USCG.shtm.

- U.S. Department of Labor, Mine Safety, and Health Administration. www.msha.gov.

- U.S. Department of Labor, Occupational Safety & Health Administration. www.osha. gov.

- U.S. National Guidelines for First Aid Training in Occupational Settings 2001 [Online]. Available: www.NGFATOS.net [3-Mar-05].

This material has been reviewed and approved by ASHI's President's Committee. The President's Committee is responsible for assuring that educational programs that carry the ASHI name or logo meet ASHI's principle objectives. President's Committee Members at time of publication include Barbara Aehlert RN, Steve Donelan, Brad Dykens EMT-P, Sue Leahy EMT, John Mateus EMT, Marcy Thobaben LPN/NREMT-B, Stephen Thomas EMT-P, and Howard A. Werman MD.

ASHI offers training and certification programs in emergency care and occupational safety and health for corporate America, government agencies, and emergency responders. To learn more about ASHI, visit www.ashinstitute.org.

ASHI has used reasonable effort to provide up-to-date, accurate information that conforms to generally accepted recommendations at the time of publication. Science and technology are constantly creating new knowledge and practice. Like any printed material, this publication may become out of date over time. Guidelines for safety recommendations for treatment cannot be given that will apply in all cases as the circumstances of each incident often vary widely. *These recommendations supersede recommendations made in previous ASHI programs.*

Alert emergency medical services (EMS) or activate your emergency action plan immediately if you are not sure an emergency exists or when any victim is unresponsive, badly hurt, looks or acts very ill, or quickly gets worse. Signs and symptoms may be incomplete and can vary from person to person. Do not use the information in this program as a substitute for professional evaluation and diagnosis from an appropriately qualified and licensed physician or other health care provider. Local or organizational physician-directed practice protocols may supersede recommendations in this program.

Municipal, state, provincial, national, or federal regulations are governmental orders having the force of law. In the United States, Canada, and most other industrialized countries, workplace safety regulations and occupational licensing requirements prescribe scope of practice, rules, standards, and conditions that every training agency, program, instructor, and licensed person must comply with. ASHI training centers and their authorized instructors must be completely familiar with the regulations and licensing requirements of persons to whom they offer training and certification. Training centers and authorized instructors must not advertise, represent, or otherwise promote that their programs will meet specific regulations or licensing requirements unless and until such is confirmed with the licensing authority and/or ASHI.

Infection Control Terminology. The Occupational Safety & Health Administration (OSHA) Bloodborne Pathogens Standard (1910.1030) uses the term "universal precautions" as an approach to infection control. The U.S. Department of Health and Human Services (HHS) and Centers for Disease Control (CDC) guidelines combine the term "universal precautions" and "body substance isolation" into a single set of precautions termed "standard precautions" for the care of patients in hospitals.[1] Isolation practices and terminology continue to evolve. For compliance with OSHA standards, the use of either universal precautions or standard precautions is acceptable.[2]

References

1. Guideline for Isolation Precautions in Hospitals Julia S. Garner, RN, MN, and the Hospital Infection Control Practices Advisory Committee. From the Public Health Service, US Department of Health and Human Services, Centers for Disease Control and Prevention, Atlanta, Georgia. Garner JS, Hospital Infection Control Practices Advisory Committee. Guideline for isolation precautions in hospitals. *Infect Control Hosp Epidemiol* 1996; 17:53-80, and *Am J Infect Control* 1996; 24:24-52. Available: www.cdc.gov/ncidod/dhqp/gl_isolation_ptI.html [25-Mar-06]

2. Occupational Safety & Health Administration. Hospital eTool—HealthCare Wide Hazards Module, (Lack of) Universal Precautions. Available: www.osha.gov/SLTC/etools/hospital/hazards/univprec/univ.html [25-Mar-06]

chapter 3   CPR and AED for the Community and Workplace

The American Safety & Health Institute (ASHI) is an association of professional safety and health educators providing nationally-recognized training programs across the United States and in several foreign countries. ASHI's mission is to continually improve safety and health education by promoting high standards for members, principles of sound research for curriculum development, and the professional development of safety and health instructors worldwide.

ASHI is a member of the National First Aid Science Advisory Board cofounded by the American Red Cross and American Heart Association®, Inc. (AHA), and a participant in the International Committee on Resuscitation (ILCOR) 2005 International Conference on Cardiopulmonary Resuscitation (CPR) and Emergency Cardiovascular Care (ECC) Science with Treatment Recommendations, hosted by the AHA. ASHI offers training and certification programs in emergency care and occupational safety and health for corporate America, government agencies, and emergency responders. To learn more about ASHI, visit www.ashinstitute.org.

ASHI's CPR and AED program content is based upon the following science, treatment recommendations, and guidelines:

- 2005 International Consensus Conference on Cardiopulmonary Resuscitation and Emergency Cardiovascular Care Science with Treatment Recommendations hosted by the American Heart Association in Dallas, Texas, January 23–30, 2005.

Circulation 2005; 112: III-5-III-16 and *Resuscitation* Volume 67, Supplement 1, Pages S1-S190 December 2005 © 2005 International Liaison Committee on Resuscitation, American Heart Association, Inc. and European Resuscitation Council.

- 2005 American Heart Association Guidelines for Cardiopulmonary Resuscitation and Emergency Cardiovascular Care. *Circulation.* 2005; 112:IV-1–IV-211© 2005 American Heart Association, Inc.

- Other evidence-based treatment recommendations or sources are referenced by endnote.

This material has been reviewed and approved by ASHI's President's Committee. The President's Committee is responsible for assuring that educational programs that carry the ASHI name or logo meet ASHI's principle objectives. President's Committee Members at time of publication include Barbara Aehlert RN, Steve Donelan, Brad Dykens EMT-P, Sue Leahy EMT, John Mateus EMT, Marcy Thobaben LPN/NREMT-B, Stephen Thomas EMT-P, and Howard A. Werman MD.

ASHI has used reasonable effort to provide up-to-date, accurate information that conforms to generally accepted treatment recommendations at the time of publication. Science and technology are constantly creating new knowledge and practice. Like any printed material, this publication may become out of date over time. Guidelines for safety recommendations for treatment cannot be given that will apply in all cases as the circumstances of each incident often vary widely. *These recommendations supersede recommendations made in previous ASHI programs.*

Alert emergency medical services (EMS) or activate your emergency action plan immediately if you are not sure an emergency exists or when any victim is unresponsive, badly hurt, looks or acts very ill, or quickly gets worse. Signs and symptoms may be incomplete and can vary from person to person. Do not use the information in this program as a substitute for professional evaluation, diagnosis, and treatment from an appropriately qualified and licensed physician or other health care provider. Local or organizational physician-directed practice protocols may supersede treatment recommendations in this program.

Municipal, state, provincial, national, or federal regulations are governmental orders having the force of law. In the United States, Canada, and most other industrialized countries, workplace safety regulations and occupational licensing requirements prescribe scope of practice, rules, standards, and conditions with which every training agency, program, instructor, and licensed person must comply. ASHI training centers and their authorized instructors must be completely familiar with the regulations and licensing requirements of persons to whom they offer training and certification. Training centers and authorized instructors must not advertise, represent, or otherwise promote that their programs will

meet specific regulations or licensing requirements unless and until such is confirmed with the licensing authority and/or ASHI.

Infection Control Terminology. The Occupational Safety & Health Administration (OSHA) Bloodborne Pathogens Standard (1910.1030) uses the term "universal precautions" as an approach to infection control. The U.S. Department of Health and Human Services (HHS) and Centers for Disease Control (CDC) guidelines combine the term "universal precautions" and "body substance isolation" into a single set of precautions termed "standard precautions" for the care of patients in hospitals.[1] Isolation practices and terminology continue to evolve. For compliance with OSHA standards, the use of either universal precautions or standard precautions is acceptable.[2]

References

1. Guideline for Isolation Precautions in Hospitals Julia S. Garner, RN, MN, and the Hospital Infection Control Practices Advisory Committee. From the Public Health Service, US Department of Health and Human Services, Centers for Disease Control and Prevention, Atlanta, Georgia. Garner JS, Hospital Infection Control Practices Advisory Commitee. Guideline for isolation precautions in hospitals. *Infect Control Hosp Epidemiol* 1996; 17:53-80, and *Am J Infect Control* 1996; 24:24-52. Available: www.cdc.gov/ncidod/dhqp/gl_isolation_ptI.html [25-Mar-06]

2. Occupational Safety & Health Administration. Hospital eTool - HealthCare Wide Hazards Module, (Lack of) Universal Precautions. Available: www.osha.gov/SLTC/etools/hospital/hazards/univprec/univ.html [25-Mar-06]

chapter 4   CPR and AED for Professionals

The American Safety & Health Institute (ASHI) is an association of professional safety and health educators providing nationally-recognized training programs across the United States and in several foreign countries. ASHI's mission is to continually improve safety and health education by promoting high standards for members, principles of sound research for curriculum development, and the professional development of safety and health instructors worldwide.

ASHI is a member of the National First Aid Science Advisory Board cofounded by the American Red Cross and American Heart Association®, Inc. (AHA), and a participant in the International Committee on Resuscitation (ILCOR) 2005 International Conference on Cardiopulmonary

Resuscitation (CPR) and Emergency Cardiovascular Care (ECC) Science with Treatment Recommendations, hosted by the AHA.

ASHI's CPR and AED program content is based upon the following science, treatment recommendations, and guidelines:

- 2005 International Consensus Conference on Cardiopulmonary Resuscitation and Emergency Cardiovascular Care Science with Treatment Recommendations hosted by the American Heart Association in Dallas, Texas, January 23–30, 2005. *Circulation* 2005; 112: III-5-III-16 and *Resuscitation* Volume 67, Supplement 1, Pages S1-S190 December 2005 © 2005 International Liaison Committee on Resuscitation, American Heart Association, Inc., and European Resuscitation Council.

- 2005 American Heart Association Guidelines for Cardiopulmonary Resuscitation and Emergency Cardiovascular Care. *Circulation.* 2005; 112:IV-1–IV-211© 2005 American Heart Association, Inc.

- Other evidence-based treatment recommendations or sources are referenced by endnote.

This program material has been reviewed and approved by ASHI's President's Committee. The President's Committee is responsible for assuring that educational programs that carry the ASHI name or logo meet ASHI's principle objectives. President's Committee Members at time of publication include Barbara Aehlert RN, Steve Donelan, Brad Dykens EMT-P, Sue Leahy EMT, John Mateus EMT, Marcy Thobaben LPN/NREMT-B, Stephen Thomas EMT-P, and Howard A. Werman MD.

ASHI offers training and certification programs in emergency care and occupational safety and health for corporate America, government agencies, and emergency responders. To learn more about ASHI, visit www.ashinstitute.org.

ASHI has used reasonable effort to provide up-to-date, accurate information that conforms to generally accepted treatment recommendations at the time of publication. Science and technology are constantly creating new knowledge and practice. Like any printed material, this publication may become out of date over time. Guidelines for safety recommendations for treatment cannot be given that will apply in all cases as the circumstances of each incident often vary widely. *These recommendations supersede recommendations made in previous ASHI programs.*

Alert emergency medical services (EMS) or activate your emergency action plan immediately if you are not sure an emergency exists or when any patient is unresponsive, badly hurt, looks or acts very ill, or quickly gets worse. Signs and symptoms may be incomplete and can vary from person to person. Do not use the information in this program as a substitute for professional evaluation, diagnosis, and treatment from an appropriately qualified and licensed physician or other health care provider. Local or organizational physician-directed practice protocols may supersede treatment recommendations in this program.

Municipal, state, provincial, national, or federal regulations are governmental orders having the force of law. In the United States, Canada, and most other industrialized countries, workplace safety regulations and occupational licensing requirements prescribe scope of practice, rules, standards, and conditions that every training agency, program, instructor and licensed person must comply with. ASHI training centers and their authorized instructors must be completely familiar with the regulations and licensing requirements of persons to whom they offer training and certification. Training centers and authorized instructors must not advertise, represent, or otherwise promote that their programs will meet specific regulations or licensing requirements unless and until such is confirmed with the licensing authority and/or ASHI.

Joint Commission on Accreditation of Healthcare Organizations (JCAHO). JCAHO Resuscitation Standard (revised PC.9.30, EP 4 effective July 1, 2006) requires that resuscitation services are available throughout the hospital. "Elements of Performance" for PC.9.30 include the requirement that "an evidence-based training program(s) is used to train appropriate staff to recognize the need for and use of designated equipment and techniques in resuscitation efforts." JCAHO defines evidence-based as "based on empirical evidence or in the absence of empirical evidence, expert consensus (such as consensus statements promoted by professional societies)." ASHI's *CPRPro for the Professional Rescuer* meets JCAHO's requirements for PC.9.30. For questions related to JCAHO standards, visit www.jointcommission.org or contact the Standards Interpretation Group at 630-792-5900.

Infection Control Terminology. The Occupational Safety & Health Administration (OSHA) Bloodborne Pathogens Standard (1910.1030) uses the term "universal precautions" as an approach to infection control. The U.S. Department of Health and Human Services (HHS) and Centers for Disease Control (CDC) guidelines combine the term "universal precautions" and "body substance isolation" into a single set of precautions termed "standard precautions" for the care of patients in hospitals.[1] Isolation practices and terminology continue to evolve. For compliance with OSHA standards, the use of either universal precautions or standard precautions is acceptable.[2]

References

1. Guideline for Isolation Precautions in Hospitals Julia S. Garner, RN, MN, and the Hospital Infection Control Practices Advisory Committee. From the Public Health Service, US Department of Health and Human Services, Centers for Disease Control and Prevention, Atlanta, Georgia. Garner JS, Hospital Infection Control Practices Advisory Commitee. Guideline for isolation precautions in hospitals. *Infect Control Hosp Epidemiol* 1996; 17:53-80, and *Am J Infect Control* 1996; 24:24-52. Available: www.cdc.gov/ncidod/dhqp/gl_isolation_ptI.html [25-Mar-06]

2. Occupational Safety & Health Administration. Hospital eTool - HealthCare Wide Hazards Module, *(Lack of) Universal Precautions.* Available: www.osha.gov/SLTC/etools/hospital/hazards/univprec/univ.html [25-Mar-06]

chapter 5   Emergency Oxygen

The American Safety & Health Institute (ASHI) is a member of the National First Aid Science Advisory Board cofounded by the American Red Cross and American Heart Association®, Inc., and a contributor to the 2005 Consensus of First Aid Science and Recommendations.

The recommendations presented in chapter 5 for emergency oxygen administration are based upon standards, guidelines, regulations, and recommendations from the following sources:

- ASTM International Standard F 2171-02 *"Standard Guideline Defining the Performance of First Aid Providers in Occupational Settings"* April 2002
- National Guidelines for First Aid Training in Occupational Settings: Guidelines for a first aid oxygen administration enrichment program
- National First Aid Science Advisory Board: American Heart Association and the American National Red Cross
- Compressed Gas Association
- U.S. Department of Transportation

ASHI offers training and certification programs in emergency care and occupational safety and health for corporate America, government agencies, and emergency responders. To learn more about ASHI, visit www.ashinstitute.org.

ASHI has used reasonable effort to provide up-to-date, accurate information that conforms to generally accepted recommendations at the time of publication. Science and technology are constantly creating new knowledge and practice. Like any printed material, this publication may become out of date over time. Guidelines for safety and recommendations for treatment cannot be given that will apply in all cases as the circumstances of each incident often vary widely. *These recommendations supersede recommendations made in previous ASHI programs.*

Alert emergency medical services (EMS) or activate your emergency action plan immediately if you are not sure an emergency exists or when any victim is unresponsive, badly hurt, looks or acts very ill, or quickly gets worse. Signs and symptoms may be incomplete and can vary from person to person. Do not use the information in this program as a substitute for professional evaluation and diagnosis from an appropriately qualified and licensed physician or other health care provider. Local or organizational physician-directed practice protocols may supersede recommendations in this program.

Municipal, state, provincial, national, or federal regulations are governmental orders having the force of law. In the United States, Canada, and most other industrialized countries, workplace safety regulations and occupational licensing requirements prescribe scope of practice, rules, standards, and conditions that every training agency, program, instructor, and licensed person must comply with. ASHI training centers and their authorized instructors must be completely familiar with the regulations and licensing requirements of persons to whom they offer training and certification. Training centers and authorized instructors must not advertise, represent, or otherwise promote that their programs will meet specific regulations or licensing requirements unless and until such is confirmed with the licensing authority, and/or ASHI.

introduction

You are reading this book because, as part of your job, you need to know more about how to aid people in medical emergencies. Whether you are a lifeguard or other professional who is required to be certified in CPR and first aid or you just need to be prepared for emergencies, this book and the accompanying online course will help you learn the basics of providing emergency care.

Complete Emergency Care is the student textbook for the following American Safety & Health Institute courses:

- Bloodborne Pathogens
- Basic First Aid for the Community and Workplace
- CPR/AED for the Community and Workplace
- CPR Pro for the Professional Rescuer
- Emergency Oxygen Administration

These may be taught separately or be combined to create an emergency care course that can be taught to anyone who needs to provide CPR as part of their official job duties or on a volunteer basis. Each chapter of this text corresponds to one of the courses.

Chapter 1 introduces you to the Occupational Safety & Health Administration standards for **bloodborne pathogens,** the diseases they can cause, and the precautions you should take to avoid becoming ill or spreading the pathogens. You'll also learn how to prevent exposure to pathogens at work by using engineering and work practice controls, following universal precautions, and wearing personal protective equipment. Finally, you'll find out what to do in case you are exposed to bloodborne pathogens and what follow-up evaluation should be done. You need to learn about bloodborne pathogens first, because your involvement in any emergency situation may put you and others at risk of contamination.

Chapter 2 presents **first aid** for many different types of medical emergencies. First, you'll receive guidance on how to deal with the legal and emotional challenges you may face when you have to provide first aid to seriously ill or injured victims. Then you'll learn how to respond when you first approach a victim and how to handle sudden illnesses, especially those that may be life threatening, and illnesses and injuries due to extreme heat or cold. You'll also learn how to provide aid for common soft-tissue injuries and injuries to the limbs, spine, and head.

Chapters 3 and **4** offer instruction on how to perform **rescue breathing** and **cardiopulmonary resuscitation (CPR).** Chapter 3 explains procedures for laypeople who want to know this skill in case they become involved in a first aid situation that requires it. Chapter 4 is for professionals whose jobs require that they be certified in CPR. Both chapters first describe stroke, sudden cardiac arrest, and the chain of survival for adults and children, then they walk you through the steps to administering rescue breathing or CPR and using an automated external defibrillator (AED). Instructions on how to aid victims of choking are also included. A brief discussion of the psychological and legal aspects of providing CPR and how to handle CPR under special conditions ends the chapters.

Chapter 5 covers the **administration of emergency oxygen** to victims. Emergency oxygen can improve the condition of all victims with serious medical problems, and we'll talk about how emergency oxygen differs from medical oxygen. You'll learn what is included in an oxygen system and how to assemble one. You'll also learn how to handle oxygen safely, how to maintain the emergency oxygen system, and when and how to provide emergency oxygen.

This text, which may be combined with an online course, will help ensure that you learn the necessary information and procedures so that you can help victims of medical emergencies.

You also will need to participate in classroom training with an instructor in order to ensure you master the needed skills.

Regardless of why you are reading this book and taking this course, you will find yourself better equipped to assist victims of medical emergencies once you're finished. You will then have the ability to help relieve victims' pain, prevent permanent injury, and perhaps even save lives. We hope that after taking this course you will feel confident that you know how to handle whatever emergency situations you encounter.

Bloodborne Pathogens

The material in this chapter will help both you and your employer to comply with the information and training aspects of the U.S. Department of Labor, Occupational Safety, & Health Administration (OSHA) bloodborne pathogens standard. For a copy of the regulatory text of the standard and an explanation of its contents, go to OSHA's Web site at www.osha.gov (search using the key words *bloodborne pathogens 1910.1030*). This text will also be available as a PDF file in the online courses.

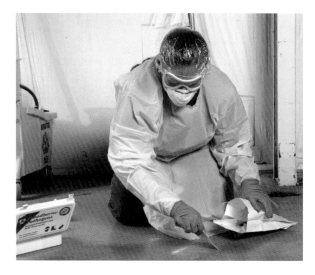

In this chapter on bloodborne pathogens, you will learn the following:

- What the bloodborne pathogens standard is and whom it covers
- What pathogens and other potentially infectious materials are
- The incidence, signs and symptoms, methods of transmission, and prevention for hepatitis B, hepatitis C, and HIV
- How to prevent occupational exposure, what an exposure control plan is, and what engineering and work practice controls are
- What universal precautions are
- What personal protective equipment is and the types available
- What to do in case of exposure and what evaluation must be done after an incident of exposure

American Safety & Health Institute (ASHI) certification may be issued only when an ASHI-authorized instructor verifies you have successfully completed the required objectives of this training program. By itself, this chapter does not constitute complete training.

Bloodborne Pathogens Standard

OSHA estimates that 8 million workers in the United States in the health care industry and related occupations are at risk of occupational exposure to bloodborne pathogens.[1] **Occupational exposure to blood or other potentially infectious materials (OPIM) puts you at risk for serious illness or death.** The viruses of the most concern are the hepatitis B virus (HBV), hepatitis C virus (HBC), and human immunodeficiency virus (HIV).

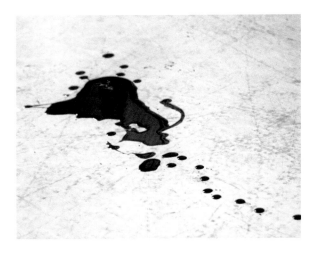

The OSHA standard requires that employers ensure that all employees with occupational exposure to bloodborne disease participate in a training program provided during working hours at no cost to the employees. Employers must also ensure that their workers receive regular training that covers the dangers of bloodborne pathogens, safety and prevention practices, and postexposure procedures. Employers must offer this training at least annually.

The hazard of exposure to infectious materials affects employees in many types of employment and is not restricted to the health care industry. Any employee who has a reasonable anticipation of contact with blood or OPIM as a result of performing his or her job duties is included within the scope of the standard. Jobs that have the potential for occupational exposure include the following:

- Physicians, physician's assistants, nurses, nurse practitioners, and other health care employees in clinics and physicians' offices

- Employees of clinical and diagnostic laboratories
- Housekeepers in health care and other facilities
- Personnel in hospital laundries or commercial laundries that service health care or public safety institutions
- Personnel in tissue banks
- Employees in blood banks
- Employees in freestanding clinics
- Employees in clinics in industrial, educational, and correctional facilities
- Employees designated to provide emergency first aid
- Dentists, dental hygienists, dental assistants, and dental laboratory technicians
- Staff of institutions for the developmentally disabled
- Hospice employees
- Home health care workers
- Staff of nursing homes and long-term care facilities
- Employees of funeral homes and mortuaries
- Employees handling regulated waste
- Custodial workers required to clean up devices or materials contaminated with blood or OPIM
- Personnel in medical equipment service and repair
- Emergency medical technicians, paramedics, and other emergency medical service providers
- Firefighters, law enforcement personnel, and correctional officers
- Maintenance workers

Accidents and unexpected illness can occur in any workplace, and exposure to blood is a possibility in all working environments. Many worksites have employees who are expected to render first aid as part of their job duties. These employees are covered by the bloodborne pathogens standard. Additionally, an employee who

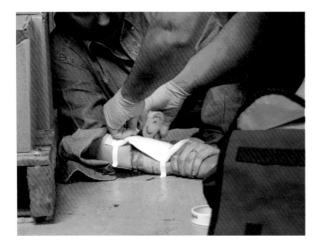

routinely provides first aid to other employees with the knowledge of the employer may be covered by the standard even if the employer has not officially designated the employee as a first aid provider.[2]

However, if an employee provides first aid or CPR as a Good Samaritan and not as a formally trained first aid provider who has been designated by the employer to give first aid, the employee is not covered by the standard.[3] Still, employers are encouraged to offer follow-up procedures for any employee who has an incident of exposure.

Bloodborne Pathogens and OPIM

Both blood and other potentially infectious materials (OPIM) may contain bloodborne pathogens. Bloodborne pathogens are bacteria and viruses present in the blood and body fluids of an infected person that can cause disease to others.

Bloodborne pathogens include, but are not limited to, the following viruses:

- Hepatitis B virus (HBV)
- Hepatitis C virus (HCV)
- Human immunodeficiency virus (HIV)

OPIM include the following:

1. Human body fluids:
   - Seminal (fluid from the male genitals)
   - Vaginal (fluid from the female genitals)
   - Cerebrospinal (fluid surrounding spinal cord and brain)
   - Synovial (fluid that lubricates joint surfaces)
   - Pleural (fluid lining the lungs and chest cavity)
   - Pericardial (fluid surrounding the heart)
   - Peritoneal (fluid contained in the abdomen)
   - Amniotic (fluid that protects the fetus throughout pregnancy)
   - All body fluids in situations where it is difficult or impossible to differentiate between body fluids

2. Any unfixed human tissue or organ (other than intact skin) from a living or dead human (e.g., laboratory tissue specimens)

3. HIV-containing cell or tissue cultures, organ cultures, and HIV- or HBV-containing culture medium or other solutions; and blood, organs, or other tissues from laboratory animals infected with HIV or HBV

Feces, nasal secretions, saliva, sputum, sweat, tears, urine, and vomit are not considered potentially infectious for bloodborne pathogens unless they are visibly bloody.[4] Still, you should take precautions, assuming that all body fluids are potentially infectious, to reduce the potential for exposure to other microorganisms that can cause other types of infections.

Hepatitis B Virus (HBV)

HBV[5,6] is a serious disease caused by a virus that attacks and causes inflammation of the liver. It can cause lifelong infection, scarring of the liver, liver cancer, liver failure, and death.

Incidence	• Number of new infections per year has declined from an average of 260,000 in the 1980s to about 60,000 in 2004. • Highest rate of disease occurs in those between the ages of 20 and 49. • Greatest decline among children and adolescents due to routine hepatitis B vaccination. • An estimated 1.25 million Americans are chronically infected, 20 to 30% of whom acquired the infection in childhood. • The percentage of cases with occupational exposure to blood is now approximately 0.5% after widespread hepatitis B vaccination of health care workers.
Signs and symptoms	• Jaundice (yellowing of skin) • Fatigue • Abdominal pain • Loss of appetite • Nausea, vomiting • Joint pain **Note:** About 30% of infected people have no signs or symptoms. Signs and symptoms are less common in children than adults.

Transmission	• Occurs when blood from an infected person enters the body of an uninfected person.
	• HBV is spread through having sex with an infected person without using a condom, by injecting drugs with shared needles, through needle sticks or exposures to sharps[a] on the job, or from an infected mother to her baby during birth.
	• People at risk for HBV infection might also be at risk for infection with hepatitis C virus (HCV) or HIV.
	• You **cannot** get HBV from these practices or sources:
	  - Sneezing or coughing
	  - Kissing or hugging
	  - Sharing eating utensils or drinking glasses
	  - Breast-feeding
	  - Food or water
	  - Casual contact (such as an office setting)

Prevention	• Hepatitis B vaccine is the best protection. • If you are having sex, but not with one steady partner, use latex condoms correctly every time you have sex. Proper use may reduce transmission. • If you are pregnant, you should get a blood test for hepatitis B. • Do not inject drugs. Never share drugs, needles, or syringes. • Do not share personal care items that might have blood on them (e.g., razors or toothbrushes). • Consider the risks if you are thinking about getting a tattoo or body piercing. • If you have or had hepatitis B, do not donate blood, organs, or tissue. • If you are a designated first aid provider, health care worker, or public safety worker, assume that the blood and other body fluids from all patients are potentially infectious. • Safely handle needles and other sharps. • Get vaccinated against hepatitis B.

[a] A sharp is any device having corners, edges, or projections capable of cutting or piercing the skin. This includes syringes with needles, razors, scalpels, and broken glassware contaminated with blood or OPIM. All sharps must be disposed into an appropriate sharps container.

The HBV vaccine is used to prevent infection by the hepatitis B virus. The vaccine works by causing your body to produce its own protection (antibodies) against the disease. The vaccine is made without any human blood or blood products or any other substances of human origin. The vaccine cannot give you the hepatitis B virus (HBV) or the human immunodeficiency virus (HIV).[7]

The bloodborne pathogens standard requires that an employer make the hepatitis B vaccination available after an employee has received the bloodborne pathogens training. This must be done within 10 working days of when the employee is assigned to a job with occupational exposure to blood or OPIM. An employee may decline the hepatitis B vaccination but decide to accept it at a later date. If the vaccine is declined, the employee must sign a document with the following statement:

I understand that, because of my occupational exposure to blood or other potentially infectious materials, I may be at risk of acquiring hepatitis B virus (HBV) infection. I have been given the opportunity to be vaccinated with hepatitis B vaccine at no charge to me. However, I decline hepatitis B vaccination at this time. I understand that by declining this vaccine, I continue to be at risk of acquiring hepatitis B, a serious disease. If in the future I continue to have occupational exposure to blood or other potentially infectious materials and I want to be vaccinated with hepatitis B vaccine, I can receive the vaccination series at no charge to me.

Effectiveness	• Medical, scientific, and public health communities strongly endorse using hepatitis B vaccine as a safe and effective way to prevent disease and death. • Everyone under 19 years of age should get vaccinated against hepatitis B.
Safety	• Scientific data show that hepatitis B vaccines are very safe for infants, children, and adults. • No confirmed evidence indicates that hepatitis B vaccine can cause chronic illnesses. • To ensure a high standard of safety with vaccines, several federal agencies continually assess and research possible or potential health effects that could be associated with vaccines.
Method of administration	• Vaccine is injected. • Vaccine is available only from your doctor or other authorized health care professional.
Benefits	• Hepatitis B vaccine prevents hepatitis B disease and its serious consequences, such as liver cancer. • The OSHA bloodborne pathogens standard requires that employers make the hepatitis B vaccine and vaccination series available at no cost to all employees who have occupational exposure.

Hepatitis C Virus (HCV)

HCV[8] is a serious disease caused by a virus that attacks the liver and causes inflammation. It can cause lifelong infection, scarring of the liver, liver cancer, liver failure, and death.

Incidence	• Number of new infections per year has declined from an average of 240,000 in the 1980s to about 26,000 in 2004. • Most infections are due to illegal injection of drugs. • Transfusion-associated cases occurred before blood donor screening; they now occur in less than 1 per 2 million transfused units of blood. • An estimated 3.9 million (1.6%) Americans have been infected with HCV, 3.2 million of whom are chronically infected.
Signs and symptoms	• Jaundice (yellowing of skin) • Fatigue • Dark urine • Abdominal pain • Loss of appetite • Nausea **Note:** 80% of people have no signs or symptoms.

Transmission	• Occurs when blood from an infected person enters the body of a person who is not infected.
	• HCV is spread by injecting drugs with shared needles, through needle sticks or exposure to sharps on the job, or from an infected mother to her baby during birth.
	• HCV can be spread by sex, but this is rare.
	• People at risk for HCV infection might also be at risk for infection with hepatitis B virus or HIV.
	• You **cannot** get HCV from these practices or sources:
	  - Sneezing or coughing
	  - Kissing or hugging
	  - Sharing eating utensils or drinking glasses
	  - Breast-feeding
	  - Food or water
	  - Casual contact (e.g., an office setting)

Prevention	**There is no vaccine to prevent HCV.** • If you are having sex, but not with one steady partner, use latex condoms correctly every time you have sex. Proper use may reduce transmission. • If you are pregnant, you should get a blood test for hepatitis C. • Do not inject drugs. Never share drugs, needles, or syringes. • Do not share personal care items that might have blood on them (e.g., razors or toothbrushes). • Consider the risks if you are thinking about getting a tattoo or body piercing. • If you are a designated first aid provider, health care worker, or public safety worker, assume that the blood and other body fluids from all patients are potentially infectious. • Safely handle needles and other sharps. • If you have or had hepatitis C, do not donate blood, organs, or tissue.

Human Immunodeficiency Virus (HIV) and Acquired Immune Deficiency Syndrome (AIDS)[9]

AIDS is a term that applies to the most advanced stages of HIV infection. By killing or damaging cells of the body's immune system, HIV progressively destroys the body's ability to fight off certain bacteria, viruses, fungi, parasites, and other microbes.

Incidence	• More than 900,000 cases of AIDS have been reported in the United States since 1981.
	• As many as 950,000 Americans may be infected with HIV, one-quarter of whom are unaware of their infection.
	• The epidemic is growing most rapidly among minority populations and is a leading killer of African American males ages 25 to 44.
	• AIDS affects nearly 7 times more African Americans and 3 times more Hispanics than whites.
	• In recent years, an increasing number of African American women and children are being affected by HIV/AIDS.
	• In 2003, two-thirds of U.S. AIDS cases in both women and children were among African Americans.
	• The risk of health care workers being exposed to HIV on the job is very low, especially if they take precautions, assuming that all body fluids are potentially infectious.
	• The average risk of HIV transmission after a needle puncture of the skin with HIV-infected blood has been estimated to be approximately 0.3%; after a mucous membrane exposure, it is approximately 0.09%.[10]
Early signs and symptoms	**Within a month or two after exposure to the virus, symptoms may imitate a flulike illness:** • Fever • Headache • Fatigue • Enlarged or large lymph nodes or swollen glands **The following are other symptoms often experienced months to years before the onset of AIDS:** • Lack of energy • Weight loss • Frequent fevers and sweating • Persistent or frequent yeast infections (oral or vaginal) • Persistent skin rashes or flaky skin • Pelvic inflammatory disease in women that does not respond to treatment • Short-term memory loss

(continued)

(continued)

Transmission	**These are the main ways HIV is transmitted:** • Having sex (anal, vaginal, or oral) with someone infected with HIV • Sharing needles and syringes with someone who has HIV • Exposure (in the case of infants) to HIV before or during birth, or through breast-feeding It is rare for a patient to give HIV to a health care worker or vice versa by accidental sticks with contaminated needles or other medical instruments. You **cannot** get HIV from these practices or sources: • Handshakes • Hugs or casual kisses • Toilet seats • Drinking fountains • Doorknobs • Dishes • Drinking glasses • Food • Pets • Mosquitoes or bedbugs
Prevention	**There is no vaccine to prevent HIV.** • Abstain from having sex or use male latex condoms or female polyurethane condoms. Proper use may reduce transmission. • Do not inject drugs. Never share drugs, needles, or syringes. • Consider the risks if you are thinking about getting a tattoo or body piercing. • If you are a designated first aid provider, health care worker, or public safety worker, assume that the blood and other body fluids from all patients are potentially infectious. • Safely handle needles and other sharps.

Safety and Prevention in the Workplace

Prevention of occupational exposure to blood-borne pathogens and OPIM requires a comprehensive approach including risk assessment and exposure control planning, engineering and work practice controls, and proper use of personal protective equipment (PPE). This section provides an overview of these critical elements of safety and prevention in the workplace.

Every employer who has employees with a risk of occupational exposure to blood or OPIM must perform an assessment of this risk and develop a written plan intended to eliminate or minimize the risk. The plan must be accessible whenever an employee or his or her designated representative requests it. Ask your employer where a written copy can be obtained.

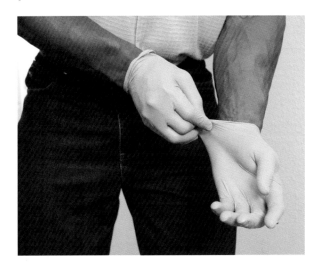

The exposure control plan must contain the following:

- **Exposure determination.** This is a list of all job classifications, tasks, and procedures with a risk of occupational exposure to blood or OPIM.
- **Schedule and method of implementation.** This is a written description of how the employer puts bloodborne pathogen compliance into practice, the employer's HBV vaccination program, what postexposure evaluation and follow-up procedures exist, and how the employer communicates bloodborne hazards to employees. Record-keeping procedures must also be addressed.
- **Documentation of consideration and implementation of appropriate commercially available and effective engineering controls designed to eliminate or minimize exposure.**
- **Procedures for evaluating the circumstances surrounding an exposure incident.**

The exposure control plan must be reviewed and updated at least annually and whenever it is necessary to reflect new or modified jobs, tasks, or procedures with occupational exposure. The exposure control plan must specify any changes in technology the employer has implemented that can eliminate or reduce exposure to bloodborne pathogens, such as safer medical devices.

The plan must also document that the employer has requested input in the identification, evaluation, and selection of effective engineering and work practice controls from employees, particularly front-line health care workers who are responsible for providing patient care. Employers must train employees to use any new devices and procedures and document this training in the exposure control plan.

Engineering and Work Practice Controls

Engineering controls are equipment or devices that help reduce exposure to potential hazards either by isolating the hazard or by removing it from the work environment. Needle disposal containers, self-sheathing needles, and needleless systems are examples. Warning labels and signs are another form of engineering control. Engineering controls must be examined and maintained or replaced on a regular schedule to ensure their effectiveness.

Work practice controls are procedures that reduce the likelihood of exposure by altering the manner in which a task is performed. Washing hands, using personal protective equipment (PPE), and decontaminating equipment or surfaces are examples of work practice controls.

Signs and Warning Labels

Signs and warning labels must be attached to all containers that are used to store, transport, or ship blood or OPIM. The containers must be either marked with a biohazard symbol or placed in a color-coded container such as a red bag.

Always place contaminated sharps in a closable, appropriately labeled or color-coded, puncture-resistant, and leakproof container immediately or as soon as possible after use.

Hand Hygiene

Hand washing[11] is one of the most important and easy work practices used in preventing the transmission of bloodborne pathogens. Wash your hands or other exposed skin thoroughly as soon as possible after an exposure incident and after removal of gloves or other personal protective equipment. Employers must provide hand-washing facilities that are readily accessible to employees. When that is not possible, employers must provide either an appropriate antiseptic hand cleanser or antiseptic towelettes.

OSHA provides a model exposure control plan that includes all the elements required by the standard in an easy-to-use template. Search for OSHA publication 3186-06N (2003) at www.osha.gov.

The Centers for Disease Control and Prevention (CDC) recommend routinely decontaminating hands with an alcohol-based hand rub. Alcohol-based hand rubs are more effective than soap and water in reducing bacteria on hands, and they cause less skin irritation.[12] If an alcohol-based hand rub is not available, or your hands are visibly soiled with blood or OPIM, wash with either a nonantimicrobial soap and water or an antimicrobial soap and water. See Skill Guide 1 on page 11 for recommended technique.

The following are additional recommendations:

- Do not wear artificial fingernails or extenders when you are in direct contact with people at high risk.
- Keep natural fingernail tips less than .25 inch (less than .6 centimeter) long.
- Remove gloves after caring for someone. Do not wear the same pair of gloves for the care of more than one person, and do not wash gloves between uses with different people.
- Change gloves as you provide care to someone if moving from a contaminated body site to a clean body site

Decontamination

Decontamination is the use of physical or chemical means to remove, inactivate, or destroy bloodborne pathogens on a surface or item to the point where the pathogens are no longer capable of transmitting infectious particles and the surface or item is rendered safe for handling, use, or disposal.

OSHA requires that equipment and surfaces be cleaned and disinfected after contact with blood or OPIM. First, clean up gross contamination with a soap-and-water solution to ensure that the appropriate disinfectant used is completely effective. All spills of blood or OPIM must be immediately contained and cleaned up by professionals or properly trained staff. See Skill Guide 2 on page 12 for recommended technique.

Appropriate disinfectants include a fresh solution of diluted household bleach. Dilute .25 cup (49.1 milliliters) of household bleach (5.25% sodium hypochlorite) in 1 gallon (3.8 liters) of cool water. A bleach-and-water solution loses its strength and is weakened by heat and sunlight. Therefore, mix a fresh bleach solution every day for maximum effectiveness. Discard any leftover bleach solution at the end of the day.[13] Contact time for bleach is generally considered to be the time it takes the product to air-dry. Other appropriate disinfectants are Environmental Protection Agency (EPA)-registered antimicrobial products that have been shown to be effective against certain bloodborne and body fluid pathogens, and high-level, "hospital-grade" disinfectants cleared by the Food and Drug Administration (FDA).[14,15] Because the effectiveness of a disinfectant is governed by strict adherence to the instructions on the label, disinfectants must be used according to the manufacturer's instructions. Employees must be trained in the proper use of disinfectants.

All equipment and working surfaces must be cleaned and decontaminated after contact with blood or OPIM. All protective coverings, such as plastic wrap and aluminum foil, must be removed and replaced as soon as possible if they become contaminated. Bins, buckets, cans, or similar containers that are reused and may be contaminated with blood or OPIM must be inspected regularly and decontaminated immediately or as soon as possible if they are visibly contaminated.

Handling Specific Items

Do not pick up broken glassware directly with your hands; use mechanical means, such as a brush and dustpan or tongs (forceps). Broken glass needs to be placed into an appropriate sharps container.

Handle contaminated laundry as little as possible. Place wet contaminated laundry in leakproof and color-coded or labeled containers at the location where it was used. Use normal laundry cycles and follow the washer's and detergent manufacturer's recommendations.

Hand Hygiene Techniques

Alcohol-Based Hand Rub

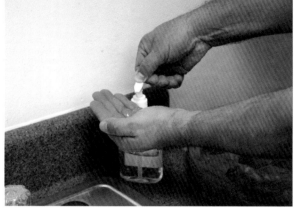

1. Apply product to palm of one hand.

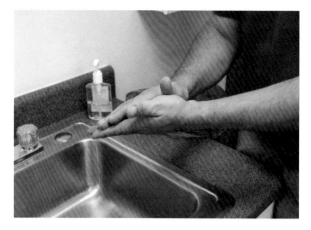

2. Rub hands together, covering all surfaces of hands and fingers, until hands are dry.

Soap and Water

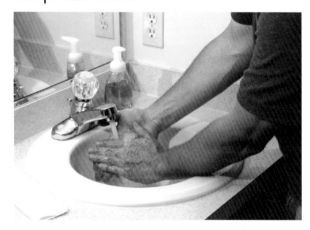

1. Wet hands first with warm water.

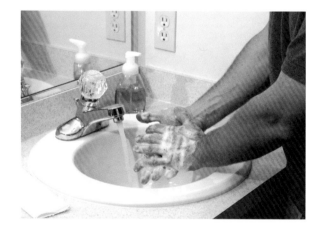

2. Apply soap to hands. Rub hands and fingers together vigorously for at least 15 seconds.

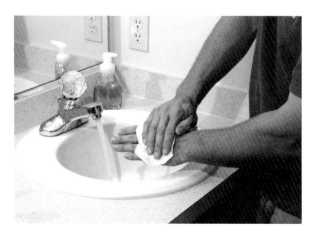

3. Rinse hands with water and dry thoroughly with a disposable towel.

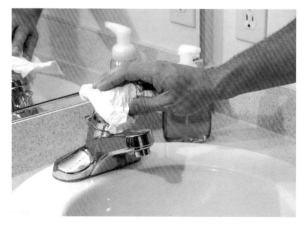

4. Use towel to turn off the faucet.

Cleanup and Disinfection of Blood or OPIM Spills

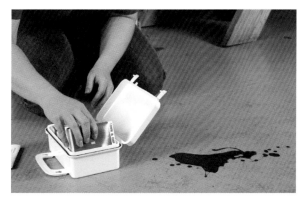

1. Locate and open spill cleanup kit.

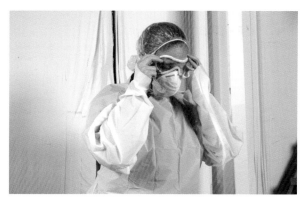

2. Put on appropriate protective clothing, including disposable aprons, caps, and eye protection.

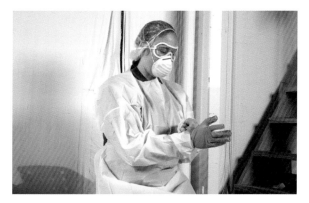

3. Wear double gloves.

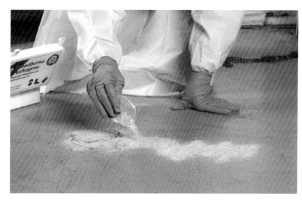

4. Pour an absorbent material over the spill.

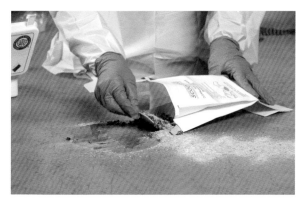

5. Use a scoop to pick up the material. Wipe up any remaining blood or OPIM with an absorbent towel. Apply a disinfectant to the area.

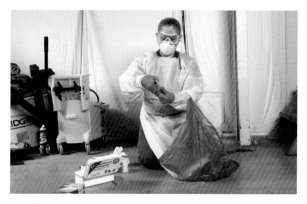

6. Place all cleanup supplies, including protective body clothing, in a red bag for proper disposal. Thoroughly wash your hands.

Universal Precautions and Personal Protective Equipment (PPE)

Universal precautions is an approach to infection control. According to the concept of universal precautions, all human blood and certain human body fluids are treated as if they were known to be infectious for HIV, HBV, and other bloodborne pathogens. To observe universal precautions means that whether or not you think the victim's blood or body fluid is infected, you act as if it is.

If blood exposure is anticipated, employers must provide appropriate PPE such as disposable gloves, gowns, laboratory coats, face shields, eye protection, pocket masks, or bag-mask devices (used for resuscitation) at no cost to employees. Employers must make certain that employees use PPE.

All PPE clothing and equipment should be of safe design and construction and should be maintained in a clean and reliable fashion. Select PPE that fits well and is comfortable to wear. Most PPE is available in multiple sizes, so take care to select the proper size. If you wear several different types of PPE together, make sure they are compatible. If your PPE does not fit properly, you may be dangerously exposed.

PPE Training

Employers are required to train each employee who must use PPE before he or she is allowed to perform any work requiring its use. The training must be documented. Employees must know the following:

- When PPE is necessary
- What PPE is necessary
- How to properly put on, take off, adjust, and wear the PPE.
- The limitations of the PPE.
- Proper care, maintenance, useful life, and disposal of PPE.[16]

Disposable Gloves

Use disposable, single-use gloves to protect your hands. Cover all cuts or sores on your hands with a bandage as additional protection before applying gloves. Inspect gloves before putting them on. If a glove is damaged, don't use it! Wearing two pairs of gloves can provide an additional barrier and further reduce the risk of transfer of bloodborne pathogens.

When taking contaminated gloves off, do it carefully. Don't snap them. This may cause blood to splatter. See Skill Guide 3 on page 14 for the recommended technique.

Never wash or reuse disposable gloves. If you find yourself in a first aid situation and you don't have any gloves handy, improvise. Use a towel, plastic bag, or some other barrier to help you avoid direct contact. Make sure there is always a fresh supply of gloves in your first aid kit.[17]

Some people are allergic to natural rubber latex, which can be a serious medical problem. Workers in the health care industry (physicians, nurses, dentists, technicians) are at risk for developing latex allergy because they use latex gloves frequently. Workers exposed to latex gloves and other products containing natural rubber latex may develop allergic reactions such as skin rashes; hives; nasal, eye, or sinus symptoms; asthma; and (rarely) shock.[18]

If you are allergic, take steps to protect yourself from latex exposure and allergy in the workplace. Taking simple measures such as using nonpowdered latex gloves and nonlatex gloves can stop the development of latex allergy symptoms and help you avoid new cases of sensitization.[19] OSHA requires that hypoallergenic gloves, glove liners, powderless gloves, or other similar alternatives be available to employees who are allergic to latex gloves.

Always place a barrier between you and a person's blood or body fluid.

Proper Removal of Contaminated Gloves

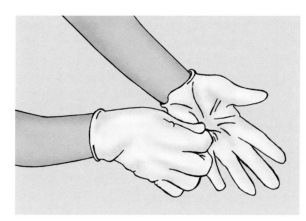

1. Without touching the bare skin, grasp either palm with the fingers of the opposite hand.

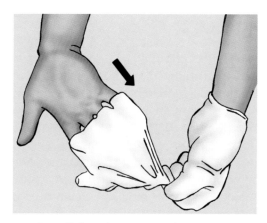

2. Gently pull the glove away from the palm and toward the fingers, removing the glove inside out. Hold on to the glove with the fingers of the opposite hand.

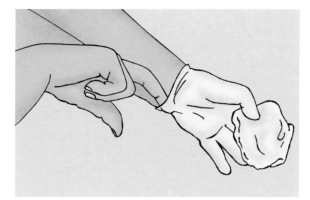

3. Without touching the outside of the contaminated glove, carefully slide the ungloved index finger inside the wristband of the gloved hand.

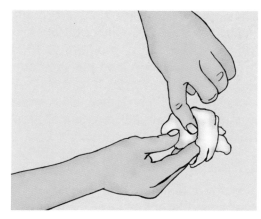

4. Gently pulling outward and down toward the fingers, remove the glove inside out.

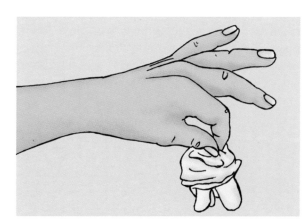

5. Throw away both gloves in an appropriate container.

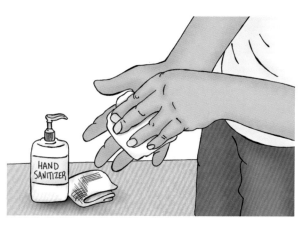

6. Use an alcohol-based hand rub to clean your hands and other exposed skin.

Eye Protection

Bloodborne viruses can be transmitted through the mucous membranes of the eyes from blood splashes or from touching the eyes with contaminated fingers or other objects. Eye protection provides a barrier to this transmission.

Goggles or glasses with solid side shields, or chin-length face shields, must be worn whenever splashes, spray, spatter, or droplets of blood or OPIM may be produced or reasonably anticipated. Appropriately fitted, indirectly vented goggles with a manufacturer's antifog coating provide the most reliable practical eye protection from blood splashes and sprays.[20] Regular prescription eyeglasses and contact lenses are not considered eye protection. Contact lenses, by themselves, offer no protection against infection.

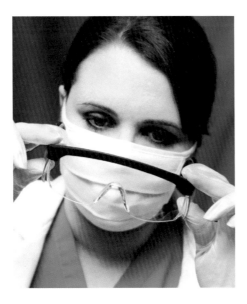

Protection During Resuscitation

Resuscitation devices (pocket masks, face shields, or bag-mask devices) must be made readily available to employees who are designated or can reasonably be expected to perform resuscitation procedures. These employees must be properly trained in the various types, use, and location of these devices according to the manufacturer's instructions or accepted medical practice. Bag-mask devices come in various sizes (see figure 1.1). It is very important to select the proper size of bag-mask device, especially for an infant or small child.

Although mouth-to-mouth breathing is a quick and effective method of providing oxygen to a person who is not breathing, emergency response

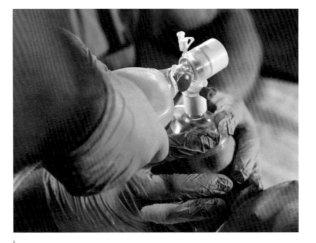

Figure 1.1 Bag-mask device.

personnel should not use unprotected mouth-to-mouth resuscitation. Equipment designed to isolate emergency response personnel from contact with the patient's saliva, respiratory secretions, vomit, blood, or body fluids should be available on all emergency vehicles and provided to all emergency response personnel who respond or potentially respond to medical emergencies or victim rescues.[21]

Protective Body Clothing

Protective body clothing such as gowns, aprons, laboratory coats, clinic jackets, surgical caps, or shoe covers must be provided at no cost to employees to prevent blood or OPIM from passing through to, or contacting, the employees' work or street clothes, undergarments, skin, eyes, mouth, or other mucous membranes. Each employer must evaluate the task and the type of exposure expected and, based on this determination, select and require the use of appropriate personal protective clothing for employees.

Contaminated PPE

Remove any PPE that becomes soiled with infectious material as soon as possible. Handle contaminated materials with caution. Place PPE that is dripping with blood or body fluids (grossly contaminated) into a container that is marked with a biohazard symbol or in a red bag. Waste containers holding contaminated PPE are considered biohazard medical waste and need to be disposed of according to individual state regulations. Discard PPE that is lightly soiled with spots of blood or OPIM in the regular trash.

Work Practices

PPE Work Practices You Should Follow

- Always wear PPE in exposure situations.
- Remove or replace any PPE that is torn or punctured or that has lost its ability to function appropriately as a barrier to bloodborne pathogens.
- Remove protective gloves before you touch noncontaminated items (such as telephones and doorknobs).
- Wear gowns or aprons, eye protection, and a mask for procedures that could involve splashing or spattering of blood or body fluids.
- Wash your hands carefully after removing protective clothing. If hand-washing facilities are not readily available, use an alcohol-based hand rub.
- If protective clothing or PPE does not fit properly, ask your supervisor or employer to provide the correct size.
- Never take contaminated protective clothing, such as lab coats, home for laundering.

General Work Practices You Should Follow

- Don't eat, drink, smoke, apply cosmetics or lip balm, or insert or remove contact lenses in areas where you could be exposed to blood or other potentially infectious materials.
- Store all food and drink away from potentially infectious materials.
- Clean and decontaminate affected work areas and surfaces thoroughly at the end of an exposure incident.

Exposure Incidents and Follow-Up

You may be exposed to blood or OPIM when you provide first aid or when you are cleaning up around your facility if syringes are discarded in the trash or on the grounds. If you have a sharps injury such as a needle stick or are exposed to blood or OPIM at work, immediately follow these steps:[22]

1. Wash cuts and needle sticks with soap and water.
2. Flush splashes to the nose, mouth, or skin with water.
3. Irrigate eyes with clean water, saline, or sterile irrigants.
4. Report the incident to your supervisor.
5. Immediately seek medical treatment.

After a report of an exposure incident (and after initial first aid), the employer must make a confidential medical evaluation and follow-up immediately available to the employee who was exposed. The evaluation and follow-up must include the following:

1. The routes of exposure and how the exposure occurred
2. Identification and documentation of the source individual,[b] unless identification is impossible or prohibited by law
3. Arrangements to have the source individual tested in order to determine if he or she is infected with HBV or HIV
4. The source individual's test results and information about laws protecting confidentiality
5. Testing of the employee's blood (after obtaining consent) as soon as possible after the exposure incident

Results of the testing must be made available to the exposed employee. The employee must be informed of all applicable laws and regulations concerning disclosure of the identity and infectious status of the individual. All medical records generated by an exposure incident must be kept confidential and may not be disclosed or reported without the employee's express written consent to any person within or outside the workplace. When postexposure vaccination for HBV or the use of antiretroviral drugs to treat HIV infection are medically indicated, administer them as soon as possible, preferably within hours.[23,24]

Employers must also make certain that a responsible person reviews the circumstances of all exposure incidents. The following factors must be documented:

1. Engineering controls in use at the time of the incident

2. Work practices followed

3. A description of the device being used (such as syringe or scalpel)

4. Protective equipment or clothing in use at the time of the incident

5. Location of the incident

6. Procedure being performed at the time of the incident

7. Employee's training

All injuries from contaminated sharps must be recorded in a sharps injury log. If necessary revisions to the exposure control plan are discovered in this process, the employer must ensure that the appropriate changes are made. The bloodborne pathogens standard requires numerous other procedures for professional evaluation, documentation, and follow-up of the circumstances surrounding an exposure incident. (See standard as directed at the beginning of this chapter.)

[b] Source individual means any individual, living or dead, whose blood or other potentially infectious materials may have been the source of exposure to the employee.

References

1. U.S. Department of Labor Occupational Safety & Health Administration. Hospital eTool—Healthcare wide hazards module: Needlesticks/sharps injuries. www.osha.gov/SLTC/etools/hospital/hazards/sharps/sharps.html. Accessed 2006 August.

2. U.S. Department of Labor Occupational Safety & Health Administration. November 27, 2001. CPL 02-02-069–CPL 2-2.69: Enforcement procedures for the occupational exposure to bloodborne pathogens. www.osha.gov. Accessed 2006 August.

3. U.S. Department of Labor Occupational Safety & Health Administration. March 23, 2001. Standard interpretations: Coverage of the BBP standard for Good Samaritan acts and personal medical conditions. www.osha.gov. Accessed 2006 August.

4. Centers for Disease Control and Prevention. Updated U.S. Public Health Service guidelines for the management of occupational exposures to HIV and recommendations for postexposure prophylaxis. *Morbidity and Mortality Weekly Report* 2005 September 30; 54 (No. RR-9). www.cdc.gov/mmwr/PDF/rr/rr5409.pdf. Accessed 2006 August.

5. U.S. Department of Health and Human Services, Division of Viral Hepatitis Centers for Disease Control and Prevention, National Center for HIV/AIDS, STD and TB Prevention. www.cdc.gov/ncidod/diseases/hepatitis/b/index.htm. Accessed 2006 August.

6. U.S. Department of Health and Human Services, Centers for Disease Control and Prevention. 2005 Hepatitis Surveillance Report No. 60. Atlanta, GA: Author.

7. National Library of Medicine. June 20, 1997. Hepatitis B vaccine recombinant (systemic). www.nlm.nih.gov/medlineplus/druginfo/uspdi/202281.html. Accessed 2006 August.

8. U.S. Department of Health and Human Services, Division of Viral Hepatitis Centers for Disease Control and Prevention, National Center for HIV/AIDS, STD and TB Prevention. August 9, 2006. Viral hepatitis C fact sheet. www.cdc.gov/ncidod/diseases/hepatitis/c/fact.htm. Accessed 2006 August.

9. Office of Communications and Public Liaison, National Institute of Allergy and Infectious Diseases, National Institutes of Health. 2005. HIV infection and AIDS: An overview. www.niaid. nih.gov/factsheets/hivinf.htm. Accessed 2006 August.

10. U.S. Public Health Service, Centers for Disease Control and Prevention. Updated U.S. Public Health Service guidelines for the management of occupational exposures to HBV, HCV, and HIV and recommendations for postexposure prophylaxis. *Morbidity and Mortality Weekly Report* 2001 June 29; 50(RR11);1-42. www.cdc. gov/mmwr/preview/mmwrhtml/rr5011a1.htm. Accessed 2006 August.

11. Centers for Disease Control and Prevention. Guideline for hand hygiene in health-care settings: Recommendations of the Healthcare Infection Control Practices Advisory Committee and the HICPAC/SHEA/APIC/IDSA Hand Hygiene Task Force. *Morbidity and Mortality Weekly Report* 2002 October 25. www.cdc.gov/mmwr/ preview/mmwrhtml/rr5116a1.htm. Accessed 2006 August.

12. Centers for Disease Control and Prevention Division of Healthcare Quality Promotion, National Center for Infectious Diseases. 2002. Hand hygiene in healthcare settings. www.cdc. gov/handhygiene/default.htm. Accessed 2006 August.

13. American Academy of Pediatrics, American Public Health Association, National Resource Center for Health and Safety in Child Care. Caring for our children. National health and safety performance standards: Guidelines for out-of-home child care, second edition. Appendix I: Selecting an appropriate sanitizer. http://nrc. uchsc.edu/CFOC/HTMLVersion/Appendix_ I.html. Accessed 2006 August.

14. U.S. Environmental Protection Agency. August 21, 2006. Pesticides: Regulating Pesticides. Selected EPA-registered disinfectants. www.epa.gov/ oppad001/chemregindex.htm. Accessed 2006 August.

15. U.S. Food and Drug Administration Center for Devices and Radiological Health. May 13, 2005. FDA-cleared sterilants and high level disinfectants with general claims for processing reusable medical and dental devices. www.fda.gov/cdrh/ode/ germlab.html. Accessed 2006 August.

16. U.S. Department of Labor Occupational Safety & Health Administration. Personal protective equipment, OSHA 3151-12R 2003. www.osha. gov/Publications/osha3151.pdf. Accessed 2006 August.

17. Tanner J, Parkinson H. Double gloving to reduce surgical cross-infection. *The Cochrane Database of Systematic Reviews* 2006 Issue 2. www.cochrane.org/reviews/en/ab003087.html. Accessed 2006 August.

18. Centers for Disease Control and Prevention National Institute for Occupational Safety and Health. NIOSH Alert. Preventing allergic reactions to natural rubber latex in the workplace. DHHS (NIOSH) publication 97-135 June 1997. www. cdc.gov/niosh/latexalt.html. Accessed 2006 August.

19. Filon FL, Radman G. Latex allergy: A follow up study of 1040 healthcare workers. *Occup Environ Med* 2006 Feb; 63(2):121-5.

20. Centers for Disease Control and Prevention National Institute for Occupational Safety and Health. 2004. Eye protection for infection control. www.cdc.gov/niosh/topics/eye/eye-infectious. html. Accessed 2006 May.

21. U.S. Department of Labor Occupational Safety & Health Administration. Bloodborne pathogens (29CFR 1910.1030) IX. Summary and explanation of the standard. www.osha.gov/ pls/oshaweb/owadisp.show_document?p_ table=PREAMBLES&p_id=811. Accessed 2006 August.

22. Centers for Disease Control and Prevention National Institute for Occupational Safety and Health. Emergency needlestick information. www.cdc.gov/niosh/topics/bbp/emergnedl. html. Accessed 2006 August.

23. U.S. Public Health Service Centers for Disease Control and Prevention. Updated U.S. Public Health Service guidelines for the management of occupational exposures to HBV, HCV, and HIV and recommendations for postexposure prophylaxis. *Morbidity and Mortality Weekly Report* 2001 June 29; 50(RR11);1-42. www.cdc. gov/mmwr/preview/mmwrhtml/rr5011a1.htm. Accessed 2006 August.

24. Centers for Disease Control and Prevention. Updated U.S. Public Health Service guidelines for the management of occupational exposures to HIV and recommendations for postexposure prophylaxis. *Morbidity and Mortality Weekly Report* 2005 September 30; 54(RR09);1-17. www. cdc.gov/mmwr/preview/mmwrhtml/rr5409a1. htm. Accessed 2006 August.

Basic First Aid

In this book, the term *basic first aid* is defined as assessments and interventions that can be performed by a bystander or by the victim with minimal or no medical equipment. A first aid provider is someone with formal training in first aid.[1] The procedures described in this chapter are intended for individuals who require or desire elementary first aid knowledge and skills for aiding both adults and children, including emergency response teams in business and industry, school bus drivers, adult residential care personnel, child care workers, teachers, parents, and babysitters. American Safety & Health Institute (ASHI) certification may be issued only when an ASHI-authorized instructor verifies you have successfully completed the required core knowledge and skill objectives of the program.

By itself, this chapter does not constitute complete training.

In this chapter you will learn the basics of first aid, which include the following:

- How to handle the legal and emotional aspects of providing first aid

- The four steps of an emergency response, including physical assessment of victims

- How to identify and treat sudden illnesses

- How to identify and treat heat- and cold-related illnesses and injuries

- How to identify and treat bleeding, shock, and injuries to soft tissue

- How to identify and treat limb, spine, and head injuries

Personal Concerns About Providing First Aid

It is frightening to be faced with a person struggling for life and not know how to help that person. The goal of first aid training is to help you avoid that situation. Correctly applied first aid can save lives. It can also reduce pain and healing time. First aid training focuses on the damaging effects of injuries and reinforces the importance

of safety. Finally, first aid training often helps to create a feeling of mutual protection and respect among co-workers and community members.

Becoming trained in first aid also means that you must deal with the legal and emotional consequences of providing first aid. Let's briefly look at these two areas.

Evidence-Based First Aid

This chapter contains evidence-based first aid recommendations. *Evidence-based* means recommendations agreed on by members of the National First Aid Science Advisory Board (NFASAB) to be safe, practical, and effective after a thorough evaluation of the medical science and recommendations based on medical literature. First aid topics and their recommendations that reflect NFASAB consensus on peer-reviewed scientific studies are followed by the letters COS, which stand for Consensus on Science. Other evidence-based recommendations and source authorities use numbered references.

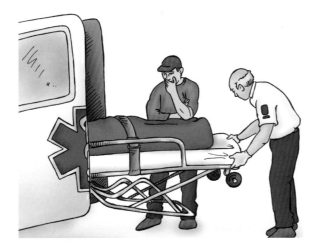

Legal Concerns

You have some legal responsibilities when you administer first aid. The following are some of the important legal principles that you need to understand.

• **Good Samaritan principle and laws.** This legal principle is based on the Biblical story of the Good Samaritan. It prevents a rescuer who has voluntarily helped a stranger in need from being sued for wrongdoing. In most parts of North America you have no legal obligation to help a person in need. However, since governments want to encourage people to help others, they pass Good Samaritan laws or apply the principle to common laws. You are generally protected from liability as long as

- you are reasonably careful,
- you act in good faith (not for a reward), and

- you do not provide care beyond your skill level.

If you decide to help an ill or injured person, you must not leave that person until someone with equal or more emergency training takes over—unless, of course, it becomes dangerous for you to stay. If your job or volunteer responsibilities include providing first aid care to others, you are not covered by Good Samaritan laws while you are working. You have a duty to respond. However, you will typically have liability protection through your employer's insurance program. Check with your employer to be sure you understand any limitations or restrictions for this coverage.

• **Consent.** Consent means permission. A responsive adult must agree to receive first aid care. Expressed consent means the victim gives his or her permission to receive care. To get consent, first identify yourself. Then tell the victim your level of training and ask if it's all right to help. *Implied consent* means that permission to perform first aid care on an unresponsive victim is assumed. This is based on the idea that a reasonable person would give permission to receive lifesaving first aid if he or she were able.

- **When caring for children,** you should gain consent from a parent or legal guardian. However, when a life-threatening situation exists and a parent or legal guardian is not available, give first aid care based on implied consent.

- **When caring for older adults,** you must keep in mind that if they are suffering from a disturbance in normal mental functioning, such as Alzheimer's disease, they may not understand your request for consent. Consent must then be gained from a family member or legal guardian. Again, when a life-threatening situation exists and a family member or legal guardian is not available for consent, give first aid care based on implied consent.

- **Preventing legal problems.** No evidence exists of a successful lawsuit in the United States against a person providing first aid in good faith. Still, it is necessary to use common sense:
  - Never attempt skills that exceed your training.
  - Don't move a victim unless his or her life is in danger.
  - If a person is weak, seriously ill, or injured or has an altered mental status, call for an ambulance immediately, even if you decide not to give first aid.
  - Always ask a responsive victim for permission before giving care.
  - Once you have started first aid, don't stop until qualified help arrives.

Emotional Concerns

Both you and the victim may suffer emotional distress during or after a traumatic incident.[2] Factors that may make such incidents more distressing include the following:

- If the incident was serious or horrible
- If the incident was caused by a person's actions, such as a bombing or mass shooting
- If the victim is a child rather than an adult

Symptoms of a traumatic stress reaction include a pounding heartbeat and fast breathing, which may begin during or within minutes of the traumatic event. Feeling guilty for not having done more, worrying about the safety of loved ones, having nightmares, and thinking about the event repeatedly may follow the incident.

Stress reactions are a normal human response to a traumatic event and are usually temporary.[3] With the help of family and friends, most people gradually feel better as time passes. If you think you need extra help coping after a traumatic event, call your doctor or ask friends if they can recommend a mental health professional. The organization you work for may have an employee assistance program available to help you.[4]

Besides attending to the legal and emotional aspects of providing first aid, you need to protect your health and the health of others by following universal precautions.

Universal Precautions

As you learned in chapter 1, universal precautions are a way to limit the spread of disease by preventing rescuers and others from having contact with blood and certain body fluids. To observe universal precautions means that whether or not you think the victim's blood or body fluid is infected, you act as if it is.

While the risk of getting a disease while giving first aid is extremely low, observing universal precautions for victims of all ages will make it lower. Be sure to wear personal protective equipment when administering first aid, such as disposable gloves and eye protection, and follow all infection-control procedures as described in chapter 1.

Emergency Response

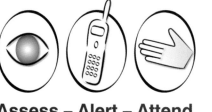

EMERGENCY ACTION STEPS

Assess – Alert – Attend to the ABCDs

The emergency action steps are the steps that you should take as you provide first aid. Follow them to respond to an emergency and manage life-threatening airway, breathing, and circulation problems in a victim of any age.

- **Assess the scene.** Whenever you recognize an emergency, assess the scene for safety. If the scene is not safe or at any time becomes unsafe, **get out!**

Roles and Responsibilities of the First Aid Provider

Roles

- Recognize the emergency and decide to help.
- Remember **safety first** (for yourself, the victim, and bystanders).
- If the victim is responsive, get his or her permission to help.
- Quickly look at and care for life-threatening conditions.
- Look for medical identification jewelry (as shown in figure 2.1) and provide care based on findings when possible.
- Continue care until someone with equal or more training takes over.
- Cooperate with your employer or public safety workers (firefighters, emergency services, law enforcement).

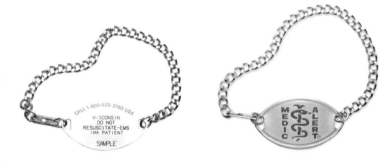

Figure 2.1 Medical ID bracelet.
Images Courtesy MedicAlert® Foundation.

Responsibilities

- Maintain composure. Do no further harm.
- Take care of your personal health and safety.
- Maintain a caring attitude.
- Maintain up-to-date knowledge and skills.
- Without putting yourself in danger, make the victim's needs your main concern.

In most cases you should not move an ill or injured person. Emergency services personnel are best trained and equipped to do this. However, in a life-threatening emergency or catastrophic disaster, you may not have time to wait for professional help. In these cases, you might have to perform an emergency move. In a situation such as a fire, explosion, or collapse, you might be able to drag a victim to safety (see figure 2.2). Drag the victim in the direction of the long axis of the body to protect the spine as best as possible. Never pull the victim sideways or pull the head away from the neck and shoulders.

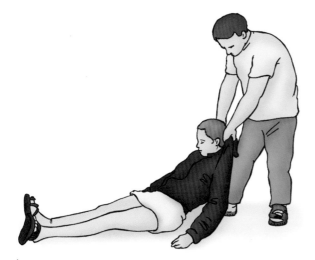

Figure 2.2   Rescue drag.

If you must perform a drag, use good lifting techniques:

- Use your legs, not your back, and keep the weight as close to your body as possible.

- Lift without twisting.

- Consider the victim's weight and the need for help.

- Know your physical ability and respect your limitations.

- **Assess the victim.** If the scene is safe, pause for a moment as you approach the victim. What is your first impression? If the victim is unresponsive or appears badly hurt, looks or acts very ill, or quickly gets worse, then begin the alert. Figure 2.3 shows an example of an emergency scene you might encounter.

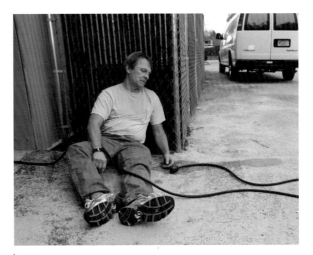

Figure 2.3   Assessing the victim.

- **Alert EMS or activate emergency action plan.** You should call 9-1-1 (or your local emergency number) to alert the emergency medical system (EMS) that you need help, or you should follow your facility's emergency action plan. An emergency action plan is a written plan that describes what actions you and other employees should take to ensure safety if an emergency occurs.

- **Attend to the victim.** Once you have alerted the proper authorities, attend to the victim's airway, breathing, and circulation (ABCs). Skill Guides 1 and 2 (pages 24-26) show how to do this for either an unresponsive or responsive victim.

Unresponsive Victim

Emergency Action Steps

Perform these steps quickly (a minute or less).

1. **Assess scene.** If the scene is unsafe or at any time becomes unsafe, **get out!**
2. **Assess victim.** Not moving? No response?
3. **Alert.** If there is no response, call EMS (9-1-1) or activate your emergency action plan.
4. **Attend to the ABCs.**

A = Airway

Open the airway. Tilt the head and lift the chin.

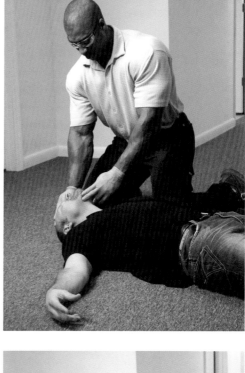

B = Breathing

- Look, listen, and feel for 5, but no more than 10, seconds.
- If the victim is not breathing normally or you are unsure, perform cardiopulmonary resuscitation (CPR; see chapters 3 and 4).
- If the victim is breathing normally, check circulation.

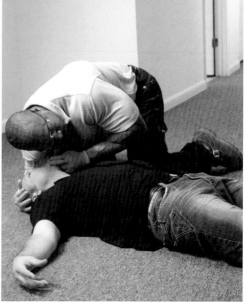

C = Circulation

- Look for blood pumping or pouring out of a wound.
- Control it with direct pressure.
- Look for normal tissue color.
- Use your exposed wrist to feel for body temperature.

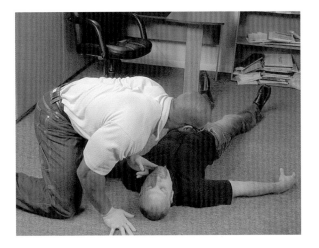

Continue to Attend to the ABCs

- Make sure the airway is open and breathing is normal.
- Control bleeding.
- Monitor tissue color and temperature.
- Help maintain normal body temperature.
- If it's available and you are properly trained, give emergency oxygen (see chapter 5).

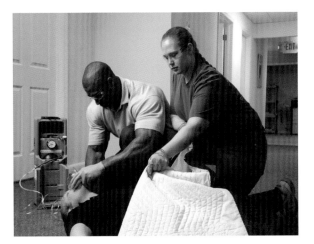

Responsive Victim

Emergency Action Steps

Perform these steps quickly (a minute or less).

1. **Assess scene.** If the scene is unsafe or at any time becomes unsafe, **get out!**
2. **Assess victim.** If the victim is responsive, identify yourself and ask if it's OK to help. If the victim appears to be weak, seriously ill, or injured, follow steps 3 and 4.
3. **Alert.** Call EMS (9-1-1) or activate your emergency action plan.
4. **Attend to the ABCs.**

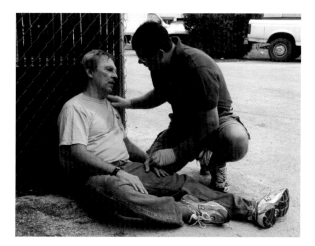

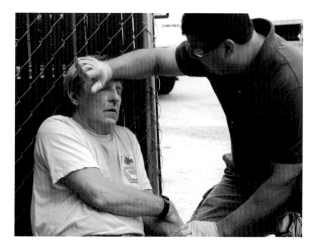

A = Airway

- Open the airway.
- Make sure the victim is fully responsive and is able to keep his or her airway open and clear.

B = Breathing

Make sure the victim is breathing normally.

C = Circulation

- Look for blood pumping or pouring out of a wound. Control it with direct pressure.
- Look for normal tissue color.
- Use your exposed wrist to feel for body temperature.

Continue to Attend to the ABCs

- Make sure the airway is open and breathing is normal.
- Control bleeding.
- Monitor tissue color and temperature.
- Help maintain normal body temperature.
- If it's available and you are properly trained, give emergency oxygen (see chapter 5).
- Consider asking about signs, symptoms, and medical history and performing a head-to-toe check for injuries (physical assessment as described in the next section).

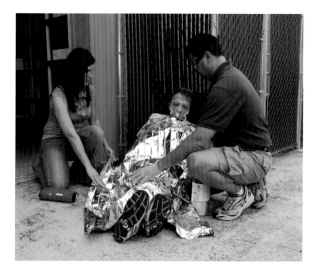

Physical Assessment

After you have assessed the victim and attended to any immediately life-threatening problems, you may want to perform a physical assessment. A physical assessment is designed to identify signs and symptoms of illness or injury not discovered when attending to the airway, breathing, and circulation. Performing a physical assessment on an injured person means doing a head-to-toe check for injuries. It also includes asking an injured or ill person about signs, symptoms, and medical history. Information obtained from performing a physical assessment can be useful for you and the victim and should be passed on to EMS providers or other health care professionals.

To conduct a physical assessment, briefly assess the body in a logical manner (head to toe). Look and feel for the signs of injury. This may be done through simple observation or by gentle touch. If the victim has been subjected to extreme forces (such as in a car crash) or you suspect head, neck, or spinal injuries, perform a head-to-toe assessment only if another first aid provider is available to help hold the victim's head still.

Assess the victim's head, neck, chest, abdomen, pelvis, and all four limbs. The acronym DOTS is helpful in remembering what to look for:

Deformities

Open injuries

Tenderness

Swelling

Ask questions to gather information about the victim's signs and symptoms and medical history. The acronym SAMPLE is helpful in remembering what information to ask about:

Signs and symptoms of injury and illness

Allergies to medications, food, and environmental conditions

Medications the ill or injured person is taking

Pertinent history of medical problems

Last oral intake of liquids or solids

Events that may have led to the illness or injury

Special Concerns for Children and Older Adults

When caring for infants and young children, reverse the head-to-toes assessment sequence so it is toes to head. Infants and young children find it threatening when strangers want to touch their face. By beginning with the toes and going backward, you reduce the chance of scaring the child. Try to gain the child's trust as you go. Be calm, friendly, and reassuring.[5]

When caring for older adults, keep in mind that talking with older adults may be difficult. Elderly victims may have trouble seeing, hearing, and talking. Speak face to face at eye level. If the older person seems confused and a relative or friend is available, check with him or her to see if this difficulty is normal for the older person. Always speak slowly, distinctly, and respectfully. Don't shout.

Recovery Positions

Recovery positions[COS] were first used in the hospital. Doctors and nurses placed an unresponsive patient on his or her side (see figure 2.4) to protect the airway from being blocked by the tongue or secretions as the person recovered after surgery. These positions are now an important skill in first aid. In the recovery position, the unresponsive victim's airway is more likely to remain open and obstructions by the

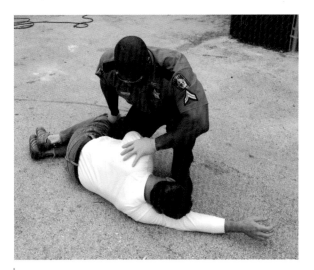

Figure 2.4 Rescuer putting victim into recovery position.

CAUTION!

Do not leave an unconscious or semiconscious person, including one passed out from excessive alcohol or drug use, alone while lying flat on his or her back. It can be fatal. If you hear gurgling or the unresponsive victim vomits, you must get the victim quickly onto his or her side to protect the airway. The victim must have an open airway in order to live!

tongue and secretions are less likely. Choking on vomit is a cause of severe brain damage and death for victims of alcohol and drug overdose. These problems may be prevented when an unresponsive victim is placed on his or her side, because fluid can drain easily from the mouth.

There are various methods of putting victims into a recovery position. No single method or position is perfect for all victims. Skill Guide 3 shows positions for an uninjured and injured unresponsive breathing victim.

For an unresponsive, uninjured victim who is breathing normally, place the person on his or her side. Be sure to do this if the victim is having difficulty with secretions or is vomiting or if you must leave the victim alone to get help.

When you place the person on his or her side, do the following:

- Make sure the victim's body position is stable so he or she does not roll onto the face or back.

- Make sure there is no pressure on the chest that could make it more difficult to breathe. Check breathing regularly.

- To prevent blood flow in the lower arm from becoming impaired, turn the victim to the opposite side if he or she is in the recovery position for more than 30 minutes.[6]

For an injured victim, don't move him or her unless you must. However, there are times when you may have to move the victim:

- When the victim is lying flat on his or her back and has debris, blood, or secretions in the mouth that might block the airway

- When you must leave the victim alone to get help

- When the victim is lying on a very hot or very cold surface and you need to get a blanket under him or her to maintain a normal body temperature

When you must place an injured person on his or her side, use a modified recovery position called the HAINES position (see Skill Guide 3). HAINES stands for **h**igh **a**rm **in** **e**ndangered **s**pine. When you use the HAINES position there is less neck movement and less risk of spinal cord damage.[7,8]

Recovery Positions

Unresponsive, Breathing Victim

Not Injured

1. Kneel beside the victim; make sure both of the victim's legs are straight.
2. Place the arm nearest to you out at a right angle to the body, elbow bent palm up.
3. Bring the far arm across the chest and hold the back of the hand against the victim's cheek nearest you.

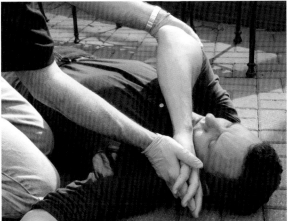

4. With your other hand, grasp the far leg just above the knee and pull it up.

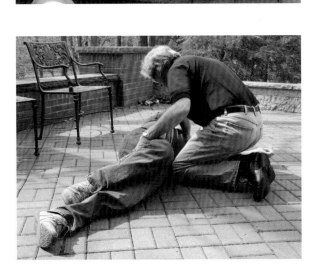

5. Keeping the victim's hand pressed against the cheek, pull on the far leg to roll the victim toward you.
6. Adjust the upper leg so both the hip and knee are bent at right angles.

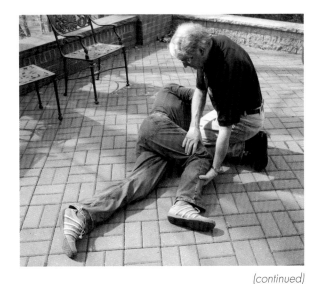

(continued)

Recovery Positions

Injured (HAINES Position)

1. Kneel beside the victim.
2. Place the victim's closest arm above the head and the farthest arm across the chest.

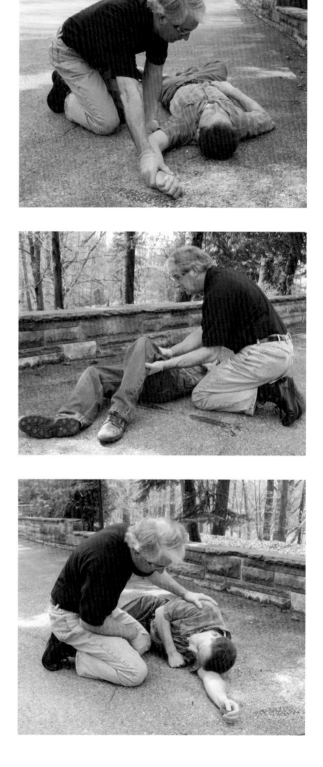

3. Bend the victim's nearest leg at the knee.
4. Place your hand under the hollow of the victim's neck to help stabilize the victim.

5. Roll the victim toward you so that the head rests on the extended arm.
6. Bend both legs at the knees to stabilize the victim.

Now that you've learned the universal first aid procedures, you can use the chart in figure 2.5 as a review. We'll now look at one more special case of first aid: aid to multiple victims.

Universal First Aid Procedures

ASSESS

- If it is not safe, or at anytime becomes unsafe, GET OUT!
- Observe Universal Precautions. Use Personal Protective Equipment!
- If victim is awake and talking, identify yourself; ask if it is okay to help.
- If victim appears weak, seriously ill or injured or is unresponsive…

ALERT

Alert EMS (Call 9-1-1) or activate your Emergency Action Plan.

ATTEND

A = AIRWAY Open Airway.	If unresponsive, tilt head – lift chin.
B = BREATHING Check Breathing.	Look, listen and feel for at least 5 seconds, but no more than 10. **UNRESPONSIVE, not breathing** – Perform CPR. **UNRESPONSIVE, breathing normally** – Place in recovery position. If injured, use HAINES position.
C = CIRCULATION	■ Look for and control severe bleeding with direct pressure. ■ Monitor tissue color and temperature. ■ Help maintain normal body temperature. ■ If it is available and you are properly trained, give emergency oxygen.

Provide First Aid Treatment
- **Suspected Spinal Injury** – Place your hands on both sides of victim's head to stabilize it.
- **Suspected Limb Injury** – Place your hands above and below the injury to stabilize it.
- Consider performing physical assessment (SAMPLE/DOTS).

Figure 2.5   Universal first aid procedures.

Multiple Victims

You may face situations in which there is more than one victim. These situations may range from automobile crashes to catastrophic natural disasters or terrorist attacks. When there are many injured victims, you must try to prioritize them by how urgently they need care. This is called *triage*, a French word meaning "to sort." The goal of triage is to do the greatest good for the greatest number. To accomplish this goal, you must not begin to provide care at random.

To begin triage, first call out, "If you can walk, come to the sound of my voice." If there are victims who can walk, instruct them to remain at a safe location. Victims who are not seriously ill or injured may also be able to help provide first aid. Now, move from victim to victim, quickly assessing their condition and sorting them into three basic groups:[9]

1. Immediate. The victim has life-threatening injuries (e.g., profuse bleeding). Rapid, life-saving treatment is urgent.
2. Delayed. The victim does not have life-threatening injuries (e.g., responsive victim with a broken leg). Treatment may be delayed.
3. Dead. No signs of life or obviously dead.

The chart in figure 2.6 provides a guide for triage.

To perform simple triage on victims of all ages:

Step 1   **Assess Victim – Assess for Responsiveness**

- If the victim is awake and responsive and not profusely bleeding, consider them "Delayed." ***Move on to the next victim.***

  If the victim is unresponsive, gently tap or squeeze their shoulder and say, "Are you okay?" If the victim does not respond;

Step 2   **A=Airway. Open Airway**

- Tilt head and lift chin

Step 3   **B=Breathing. Check for Breathing**

- Look, listen and feel for breathing
- If victim takes a breath, place them on their side in the recovery position. If injured, use the HAINES Recovery Position. ***Move on to Assess Circulation.***
- If victim does not take a breath, reposition the head to make sure the airway is open.
- If victim still does not take a breath, consider them "Dead." ***Move on to the next victim.***

  Note: The time devoted to rescue breathing and chest compressions is not justified when there are multiple victims needing first aid.

Step 4   **C=Circulation. Assess Circulation**

- Check for profuse bleeding. If present, take immediate action to stop it. If another first aid provider is available, ask them to maintain direct pressure on the wound. Consider them "Immediate."
- ***Move on to the next victim. Begin with Step 1.***

Figure 2.6   Four steps of triage.

Sudden Illness

A medical emergency can be either an injury or an illness. This section covers illnesses that can suddenly become an emergency and threaten life.

Two major sudden illnesses you may encounter are acute coronary syndromes (heart attacks) and strokes. Because first aid for these conditions is closely tied to CPR and automated external defibrillator (AED) use, their signs and symptoms and first aid treatment are discussed in chapters 3 and 4 on CPR and AED use.

A responsive victim of sudden illness usually has associated signs and symptoms. A sign is the noticeable evidence of a disease and is something you can see (such as a rash). A symptom is something the victim complains about (such as chest pain).

Note: If the victim is awake and talking, identify yourself and ask if it's OK to help. If the victim has serious warning signs and symptoms, alert EMS or activate your emergency action plan immediately.

One important sign is altered mental status. This is a sudden or gradual change in personality, behavior, or consciousness that can range from mild anxiety to inability to speak and communicate to complete unconsciousness. There are many reasons for an altered mental status, including heart problems, stroke, poisoning, overdose, diabetic problems, fever, head injury, infectious illness, low levels of oxygen in the brain, and seizures. The period of altered mental status may be brief or prolonged. **Altered mental status is a serious warning sign in both adults and children.**

Let's look at some specific sudden illnesses and conditions you may encounter.

Serious signs and symptoms for adults	Serious signs and symptoms for children
Alert EMS or follow emergency action plan immediately if the victim has any of the following: • Altered mental status • Abnormal tissue color (blue, purple, gray, or very pale) • Difficulty breathing or shortness of breath • Pain, severe pressure, or discomfort in the chest • A temperature of 105 °F (40.56 °C) or higher (heatstroke) • Appears weak, very ill, or in severe pain	Alert EMS or follow emergency action plan immediately if the child has any of the following: • Altered mental status • Abnormal tissue color (blue, purple, gray, or very pale) • Difficulty breathing or shortness of breath, persistent coughing, wheezing, or chest tightness • Seizure (in a child without a history of seizure) • Severe stiff neck, headache, and fever • A temperature of 105 °F (40.56 °C) or higher (heatstroke) • Appears weak, very ill, or in severe pain **Signs and symptoms that require medical attention within 1 hour:**[10] • Sudden onset of blood-red or purple rash[a] • Fever in a child of any age who looks more than mildly ill • Fever in a child less than 2 months (8 weeks) of age • A large volume of blood in the stool

[a] A rash is a symptom of many different kinds of childhood infectious illnesses, including chicken pox and scarlet fever. It may be triggered by other infections, such as Rocky Mountain spotted fever or ringworm.

Asthma or Reactive Airway Disease

Asthma or reactive airway disease[COS] causes the air passages in the lungs to become narrower from swelling and extra mucus. This limits airflow into and out of the lungs and causes wheezing and/or shortness of breath.

A *nebulizer* turns liquid medicine into a mist for inhaling (see figure 2.7). When victims use a nebulizer, they should follow these instructions:

1. Place the air compressor on a sturdy surface.
2. Put the medication into the nebulizer cup.
3. Assemble the nebulizer cup and mouthpiece.
4. Connect the tubing to the air compressor and nebulizer cup.
5. Turn on the air compressor.
6. Take slow, deep breaths. If possible, hold each breath for 2 to 3 seconds to help the medication get into the lungs.
7. Continue until the nebulizer cup is empty (about 10 minutes).

A *metered-dose inhaler* is a device used for inhaling a specific dose of medication as a fine spray or powder. When victims use a metered dose inhaler, they should follow these instructions:

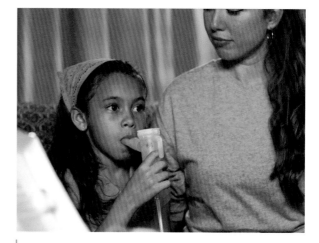

Figure 2.7   Using a nebulizer.

- Remove the cap and shake the inhaler.
- Hold the inhaler upright. Tilt your head back slightly and breathe out.
- Press down on the inhaler to release the medication and start to breathe in slowly for 3 to 5 seconds. Hold each breath for 10 seconds to allow the medicine to go deeply into the lungs.
- Repeat as directed.

Different types and brands of inhalers require different techniques (e.g., spacers, dry powder inhaler). Assist the victim with his or her medication as prescribed.

Signs and symptoms	First aid
Symptoms vary. They can be very mild to life threatening. • Constant coughing, especially worse at night and early morning • Anxiety • Sudden onset of wheezing • Chest tightness • Shortness of breath • Extreme difficulty breathing • Bluish color to lips and face • Pounding heart • Sweating • Altered mental status	If the victim is unable to administer the prescribed medication (using a nebulizer or metered-dose inhaler) without assistance, help him or her administer it.[b] **Alert EMS if the victim has any of the following:[11]** • No improvement 15 to 20 minutes after the initial treatment with medication • Constant coughing • Difficulty breathing, with the chest and neck pulled in • Stooped body posture • Struggling or gasping • Trouble walking or talking • Child stops playing and can't start activity again • Lips or fingernails are gray or blue Comfort, calm, and reassure the victim while awaiting EMS.

[b] State laws, regulations, and occupational licensing requirements may prescribe specific practices, rules, standards, and other conditions for assisting with prescribed medications.

Severe Allergic Reaction (Anaphylaxis)

Anaphylaxis[COS] is a sudden, severe allergic reaction that involves the whole body. Swelling of the lips, eyelids, throat, and tongue can block the airway. **Anaphylaxis is fatal without prompt treatment.** Anyone with a history of anaphylaxis must keep an epinephrine auto-injector on hand at all times. **Waiting for paramedics may significantly increase the risk of death.**

An *epinephrine auto-injector* is a device that allows an anaphylaxis victim to inject himself or herself with epinephrine, a substance that temporarily reverses the allergic reaction.

When victims use the auto-injector, they should do the following (see figure 2.8):[12,13]

1. Unscrew the yellow or green cap of the EpiPen or EpiPen Jr. carrying case and remove the auto-injector from the storage tube.

2. Grasp the unit with the black tip pointing downward.

3. With your other hand, pull off the gray safety release.

4. Hold the black tip near the outer thigh.

5. Swing and jab the unit firmly into the outer thigh until it clicks so that the unit is at a 90° angle to the thigh. (The auto-injector is designed to work through clothing.)

6. Hold the auto-injector firmly against the thigh for approximately 10 seconds. (The injection is now complete. The window on the auto-injector will show red.)

7. Remove the unit from the thigh and massage the injection area for 10 seconds.

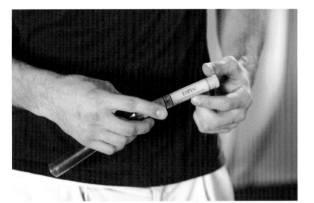

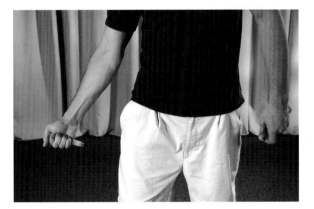

Figure 2.8 Preparing to use an epinephrine auto-injector.

Signs and symptoms	First aid
Rapid onset of the following: • Anxiety • Hives or itching • Sensation of heart pounding • Nausea or vomiting • Abdominal pain or cramping • Diarrhea • Swelling of lips, eyelids, throat, and tongue • Extreme difficulty breathing • Coughing or wheezing • Altered mental status • Blueness of skin, lips, nail beds • Complete airway obstruction	Assess, alert, and attend to the ABCs • If the victim carries a lifesaving epinephrine auto-injector prescribed by a physician, help him or her use it. If the victim is unable to use it, you should administer it. Its beneficial effect is relatively short, so the victim requires immediate medical assistance. • Comfort, calm, and reassure the victim while awaiting EMS. • **Do not** put your thumb, fingers, or hand over the black tip. • **Do not** remove the gray safety release until you are ready. • **Do not** use if the solution is discolored or a red flag appears in the clear window.

8. Call 9-1-1 and seek immediate medical attention.

9. Carefully place the used auto-injector, needle end first (without bending the needle), into the storage tube of the carrying case. Then screw the cap of the storage tube back on completely and take it with you to the emergency room.

Immediately after the victim has used the auto-injector, you should do the following:

• Direct the victim to the nearest hospital emergency room or call 9-1-1.

• The victim may need further medical attention. The victim should take the used auto-injector along.

• The victim should tell the doctor that he or she has received an injection of epinephrine in the thigh.

• The victim should give the used auto-injector to the doctor for inspection and proper disposal.

Note: Most of the liquid (about 90%) stays in the auto-injector and cannot be reused. However, you will know that a correct dose of the medication has been delivered if the red flag appears in the window.

Diabetes

Diabetes is a chronic disease characterized by an imbalance of blood sugar and insulin. A medical emergency occurs when blood sugar becomes very high or very low. Proper first aid can be lifesaving.

Type 1 diabetes is usually diagnosed in children and young adults. In this condition, the body does not produce insulin, a hormone that controls the level of glucose (sugar) in the blood. Cells cannot use glucose without insulin.

Type 2 diabetes is the more common form. In this condition, the body does not produce enough insulin or the cells ignore the insulin.

Signs and symptoms	First aid
Very low blood sugar • Pale or sweaty • Altered mental status • Anxiety or trembling • Pounding heart • May appear drunk • Hungry or weak • Fainting • Seizure • Unconsciousness **Very high blood sugar** • Altered mental status • Nausea or vomiting • Flushed, hot, dry skin • A strong, fruity breath odor • Drowsiness or difficulty waking up • Rapid, deep breathing • Unconsciousness	**Assess, alert, and attend to the ABCs** **Responsive (awake, able to swallow)** If the person is *known* to have diabetes: • Attempt to raise the victim's blood sugar level as quickly as possible.ᶜ Give him or her about 6 ounces of fruit juice. • If the person does not behave normally within about 15 minutes, call 9-1-1 or activate your emergency action plan.[14] • Comfort, calm, and reassure the victim while awaiting EMS. • **Do not** give the victim anything by mouth if the victim is unresponsive or semiconscious and unable to swallow.

ᶜ Without a medical device called a blood glucose meter, it can be difficult to tell whether the person's blood sugar is very high or very low. When you are uncertain, it is best to give sugar. The immediate effects of low blood sugar can be more harmful than those of high blood sugar. If very low blood sugar is the problem, recovery will usually occur in 10 to 15 minutes. If not, the problem may be very high blood sugar. Prompt medical treatment is required.

Seizures

A seizure is a sudden attack, usually related to excessive electrical activity in the brain. Seizures can be caused by any of the following conditions:

- Epilepsy
- Head injury
- Brain tumor
- Meningitis
- Stroke
- Very low blood sugar
- Drug use
- Alcohol withdrawal
- Very high fever
- Illness in pregnancy

Signs and symptoms	First aid
Simple = no loss of consciousness • Staring spells • Confusion • Wandering aimlessly • Strange behavior **Complex = loss of consciousness** • The victim suddenly becomes stiff and falls to the ground • Twitching or shaking of the body (convulsions) • Recovers quickly, may be confused *Most seizures happen without warning, last only a short time, and stop without any special treatment. Those known to have frequent seizures do not usually need to go to the hospital, but even mild seizures should be reported to the victim's doctor.*	**Simple** • **Do not** restrain the victim. • Guide the victim away from dangerous situations. • Comfort, calm, and stay with the victim until he or she has fully recovered. **Complex** • Stay calm and note the time. • Move objects away that the victim may strike. • Do not restrain the victim. • Allow the seizure to take its course. • Do not put anything in the victim's mouth, including your finger. The victim has no danger of swallowing the tongue. • When the seizure is over, place the victim in the recovery position. • Provide privacy to minimize embarrassment.

Poison

A poison[cos] is any substance that causes injury, illness, or death when swallowed, contacted by skin, or inhaled.

Swallowed

- Drugs (prescription, illegal, over-the-counter)
- Alcohol
- Household cleaning products
- Cosmetics
- Pesticides, paints, solvents
- Contaminated foods
- Poisonous plants (plants and plant parts can cause harm)

Skin Contact

- Corrosives (alkalis, acids, hydrocarbons)
- Poisonous plants (poison ivy, oak, sumac)

Inhaled

- Natural gas
- Carbon monoxide
- Environments contaminated with harmful dusts, fogs, fumes, mists, gases, smokes, sprays, or chemical vapors

Workplace safety regulations in the United States and other countries require appropriate training and equipment (respirators) for employees who must enter an environment that is immediately dangerous to life or health.[15]

Of the 2,395,582 human exposures to poison reported in the United States in 2003, the majority occurred at home (92.6%). The rest occurred in the workplace, including schools, health care facilities, restaurants, and other types of food service operations. Although most poisoning exposures are accidental, the majority of poisoning deaths (79%) were the result of intentional actions, primarily suicide and drug abuse or misuse.[16]

Signs and symptoms	First aid
Wide ranging and variable. Signs and symptoms of poisoning can copy those of common illnesses.	**Swallowed poison** • Call **Poison Control Center at 800-222-1222** (in the U.S.) to talk to a poison expert. • Have all medicine bottles, containers, or samples of poisoning substance available. If you go to a hospital's emergency department, take them with you. • Giving anything by mouth may be harmful. • **Do not** give the victim water or milk unless advised by Poison Control Center expert. • **Do not** induce vomiting. • **Do not** administer syrup of ipecac or activated charcoal unless advised by Poison Control Center expert. **Skin contact** Quickly remove clothing, rinse skin with large amounts of tap water. **Inhaled poison** • Assess, alert, and attend to the ABCs. • Get the victim to fresh air right away.

Emergencies During Pregnancy

Illnesses and problems can occur during pregnancy that can put both mother and child in danger.

Signs and symptoms	First aid
Serious warning signs and symptoms: • Severe abdominal pain • Persistent vaginal bleeding • Gushing amniotic fluid • Sudden severe headache • Altered mental status • Seizure • Fainting or loss of consciousness • Shock *If the victim feels faint, has signs or symptoms of shock, or is unresponsive and is more than 3 months pregnant, place her on her left side in the recovery position. When the victim is lying faceup, the baby puts pressure on a major vein that returns blood to the heart. Placing the woman on her left side reduces this pressure and provides the most blood flow to mother and baby.*	Assess, alert, and attend to the ABCs • Whenever possible, use a female first aid provider. • Have the woman assume the position that makes her most comfortable. • Get a SAMPLE history (see description on page 27). • If the woman is reluctant to discuss problems related to the pregnancy, respect her wishes. • For significant vaginal bleeding (use of more than two sanitary pads per hour), have the victim press a sanitary pad or towel to the area. • Help the victim maintain a normal temperature and do not let her become chilled or overheated. • Comfort, calm, and reassure the victim while awaiting EMS. • **Do not** examine the vagina. • **Do not** place dressings inside the vagina.

Heat- and Cold-Related Illness and Injury

Exposure to hot and humid conditions can lead to heat exhaustion and heatstroke. Exposure to cold can lead to frostbite and hypothermia. These are serious conditions that require immediate attention.

Heat Exhaustion and Heatstroke

Extended exposure to a hot, humid environment can overwhelm the body's ability to cool itself down. *Heat exhaustion* develops when the body encounters high temperatures to which it hasn't yet acclimated. In heat exhaustion the body temperature is usually less than 104 °F (40 °C).

Heatstroke is a life-threatening medical emergency. With heatstroke, the body temperature exceeds 105 °F (40.6 °C). Severe injury can result from this high body temperature, causing permanent damage to organs such as the brain and spinal cord.

It is important to recognize and to treat the symptoms of heat illness early to prevent a victim from progressing from heat exhaustion to heatstroke. **If the victim is unresponsive or has an altered mental status, alert EMS or follow your emergency action plan immediately. Begin immediate cooling with any resources available.**

Special Concerns for Children and Older Adults

Young children and the elderly with chronic diseases (or those who cannot get out of the heat) are at great risk for heatstroke and death.[19,20] First aid treatment is the same in all heat emergencies: **Cool the victim down!**

Signs and symptoms	First aid
Heat exhaustion can look like many other common illnesses. **Early** • Heavy sweating • Thirsty • Minor muscle "twitches" that progress to painful cramping[17] **Later** • Pale, cool, and moist skin • Headache • Nausea and vomiting • Weak, dizzy • Feels faint or collapses	**Assess, alert, and attend to the ABCs** **Responsive (awake, able to swallow)** • Have the victim lie down in a shady cool place. • Loosen or remove excess clothing. • Give the victim cool sport drinks (such as Gatorade) to replace lost fluid, salts, and minerals. If not available, give cool water. • Apply cool, wet cloths to the victim's skin. • Use a fan to lower body temperature. • Place cold compresses on the victim's neck, groin, and armpits.
Heatstroke can have any or all of the previously listed symptoms along with the following: • Altered mental status (confusion, hallucinations, bizarre behavior) • Hot, red, dry skin or heavy sweating • Seizure • Unconsciousness	**Assess, alert, and attend to the ABCs** • Begin cooling with any resources available. • Spray or pour water on the victim and fan him or her. • Apply ice packs to the victim's neck, groin, and armpits or cover the victim with a wet sheet. • Place the victim on his or her side in the recovery position to protect the airway. • Provide continuous cooling until EMS arrives. • With rapid cooling and medical treatment, the survival rate approaches 90%.[18] • **Do not** underestimate the seriousness of heat illness, especially if the person is a child or elderly. • **Do not** give the victim anything by mouth if he or she is vomiting or unconscious.

Prevention tips
- When working in the heat, take rest periods in a cool environment and drink plenty of fluids.
- **Never** leave a child alone in a motor vehicle in the heat, even to run a quick errand. The passenger compartment can quickly turn into a fatal oven.[21]

Frostbite and Hypothermia

Frostbite and hypothermia[COS] are the most dangerous cold-related conditions.

Frostbite develops when the skin freezes (see figure 2.9). Body parts that may be exposed to the cold are the most likely to be affected (fingers, toes, earlobes, cheeks, nose). Affected parts may need to be amputated.

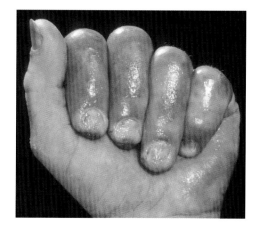

Figure 2.9 Frostbitten hand.
© SIU BioMed/Custom Medical Stock Photo.

Signs and symptoms	First aid
Frostbite **Early** • Pins and needles sensation • Throbbing **Late** • Frozen (no feeling) • Hard, pale, cold, numb skin	**Assess, alert, and attend to the ABCs** If EMS or medical attention is available: • Move the victim to a warmer place. • Remove constricting jewelry and wet clothing. • Place a sterile dressing between frostbitten fingers and toes. • Wrap frostbitten area with sterile dressings. • Comfort, calm, and reassure the victim. If EMS or medical attention is not available: • Move the victim to a warmer place. • Remove constricting jewelry and wet clothing. • Immerse the frostbitten areas in warm water (not hot) for 20 to 30 minutes. The recommended water temperature is 100 to 105 °F (38 to 40 °C). • Severe burning pain, swelling, and color changes may occur. • **Do not** rewarm if there is a chance refreezing may occur.[23] • **Do not** rub or massage the affected area. • **Do not** disturb blisters on frostbitten skin. • **Do not** give the victim alcoholic beverages. Alcohol does not help and may be harmful.
Hypothermia[COS] **Early** • Frostbite • Pale, cold skin • Weakness, loss of coordination • Altered mental status • Uncontrollable shivering **Late** • No shivering • Slow (or absent) breathing or heartbeat	**Assess, alert, and attend to the ABCs** • Get the victim indoors or out of the wind. • Remove wet or constricting clothes and replace them with dry ones. • Cover the victim with warm blankets. • Cover the victim's head and neck to help retain body heat. • Place the victim near a heat source and place containers of warm, but not hot, water in contact with the skin. • Comfort, calm, and reassure the victim until EMS arrives.

Hypothermia[COS] is a life-threatening medical emergency. In hypothermia, the body temperature has decreased to 95 °F (35 °C) or less. The following are risk factors for developing hypothermia:

• Age greater than 65
• Mental impairment
• Alcohol or drug abuse

Because of exposure to cold, a victim with frostbite frequently has hypothermia.[22] When encountering frostbite, always check for hypothermia and treat those symptoms first. **If the victim is unresponsive or has an altered mental status, alert EMS or follow your emergency action plan immediately.**

All deaths from exposure to extreme cold are preventable. Early recognition of the signs and symptoms, along with awareness of risk factors, can help minimize both injury and death.

Bleeding, Shock, and Soft-Tissue Injuries

Bleeding and shock can arise in many types of injuries and are often a concern when you are giving first aid. Other types of injuries for which signs and symptoms and treatment are described here include wounds, burns, bites and stings, dental injuries, eye injuries, and nosebleeds.

Severe Bleeding and Shock

Life cannot continue without an adequate amount of blood to carry oxygen to body tissues. The longer a victim bleeds from a major wound, the less likely he or she is to survive. Excessive bleeding[COS] will lead to shock, which results in a dangerous drop in blood flow and a lack of oxygen to body tissues. Shock will lead to death if not treated promptly.

Condition	Signs and symptoms	First aid
Severe external bleeding	• A large amount of blood is pumping, gushing, or pouring from an open wound • Pain, shock	**Apply direct pressure** • Direct pressure is considered the safest and most effective technique that can be used in the control of bleeding. • Observe universal precautions! Use personal protective equipment.
Internal bleeding	• Abdominal pain • Blood in stool, urine, vomit • Shock	**Care for shock** (see Skill Guide 4)
Shock	**Early** • Victim appears uneasy, restless, or worried **Later** • Changes in responsiveness • Cool, wet skin from heavy sweating • Pale or bluish tissue color • Shivering • Intense thirst • Nausea, vomiting • Shallow or gasping breathing • Below-normal body temperature	**Help body preserve oxygen** • Keep the airway open. • Ensure normal breathing. • Control severe bleeding. • Maintain normal body temperature. Prevent chilling or overheating. • If it's available and you are properly trained, give emergency oxygen. • It is best to leave the victim lying flat, especially when there are serious injuries to the pelvis, lower limbs, head, chest, abdomen, neck, or back.

Severe Bleeding and Shock

Emergency Action Steps

1. **Assess scene.** If the scene is unsafe or at any time becomes unsafe, **get out!**
2. **Assess victim.** If the victim is responsive, identify yourself; ask if it's OK to help. If the victim appears weak, seriously ill, or injured, follow steps 3 and 4.
3. **Alert.** Call EMS (9-1-1) or activate your emergency action plan.
4. **Attend to the ABCs.** Ensure an open airway and normal breathing, then control bleeding.

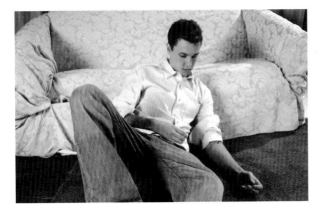

Apply Direct Pressure

- Rip or cut away the clothing so the wound can be seen.
- Place an absorbent pad directly over the wound.
- Apply firm, direct pressure over the wound.
- Victims can do this for themselves if they are able.

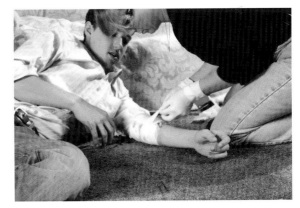

Apply Pressure Bandage

- Wrap an elastic bandage snugly over the pad to maintain pressure and hold the gauze in place.
- "Snugly" means a finger can be slipped under the bandage.

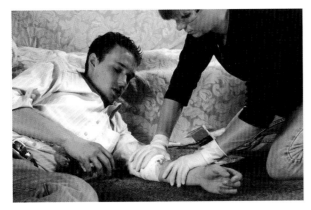

Control Bleeding

- If bleeding continues or first dressings become soaked with blood, apply more pads and dressings and maintain direct pressure.
- Do not remove the first dressings.

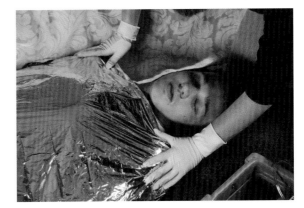

Manage Shock

- Keep the victim flat.
- Make sure the victim has an open airway and adequate breathing.
- Keep bleeding under control.
- Prevent chilling or overheating.
- If it's available and you are properly trained, give emergency oxygen.

Wounds

A wound is a break in the skin. Wounds can range from a tiny splinter to a complete amputation. All wounds need first aid, but serious wounds require medical attention. A wound also may be a sign of serious injury to deeper tissues and organs. Your role is to control bleeding, reduce pain, and prevent infection.

Major wounds	Signs and symptoms	First aid
Amputation or avulsion	Amputation is loss of a body part. Avulsion means that some tissue remains connected. • Massive or minimal bleeding may be present • Pain • Shock (pale or clammy skin, anxiety, weakness or fainting, nausea or vomiting)	**Assess, alert, and attend to the ABCs** • Control bleeding. • Care for shock. • Amputated body parts can often be reattached. If possible, get the severed part back and give it to EMS providers or take it to the hospital with the victim. • Cooling the body part will keep it alive much longer. • Wrap the severed part in a sterile or clean cloth. Place it in a tightly sealed plastic bag or waterproof container. • Place the bag or container on ice. Do not sink the part in water, and do not put it directly on ice. Chill, but do not freeze it.
Impaled object	An object embedded in tissue • Bleeding • Pain • Shock (pale or clammy skin, anxiety, weakness or fainting, nausea or vomiting)	**Assess, alert, and attend to the ABCs** • Control bleeding by applying pressure around the object. • Place bulky dressings around the object for support. • Wrap an elastic adhesive bandage over the dressing to keep pressure on it. Do not remove the object unless it is through the cheek and blocks breathing.
Open chest wound	• Bleeding • Pain • Shock (pale or clammy skin, anxiety, weakness or fainting, nausea or vomiting)	**Assess, alert, and attend to the ABCs** • Quickly check the victim to see if there are both entry and exit wounds. If there are two wounds, treat the more serious one first. • Apply direct pressure until the bleeding stops or EMS arrives. • If you see foamy, bloody air bubbles or you hear a sucking sound, immediately cover the wound with airtight materials (plastic wrap, plastic bag). The covering should be wide enough to extend 2 inches (5 centimeters) or more past the edges of the wound in all directions. This will prevent air from entering the victim's chest cavity with each breath. • If tape is available, tape three sides of the covering to the chest wall. Leave one corner of the material untaped. This allows trapped air to escape. If trapped air can't escape, the victim's lung may collapse.

Open abdominal wound	• Bleeding • Pain • Protruding objects or organs • Shock (pale or clammy skin, anxiety, weakness or fainting, nausea or vomiting)	**Assess, alert, and attend to the ABCs** • Do not attempt to remove clothing that is stuck to the wound. • Quickly check the victim to see if there are both entry and exit wounds. If there are two wounds, treat the more serious wound first. • **Do not** push organs back inside the body. • **Do not** apply direct pressure on the wound or exposed internal parts, because this could cause further injury.
Minor wounds[cos]	**Signs and symptoms**	**First aid**
Types • Abrasion • Laceration • Puncture • Incision	Break or opening in the skin • Bleeding may be minor, moderate, or severe • Bruising, pain • Protruding objects or organs • Infection • Shock (i.e., pale or clammy skin, anxiety, weakness or fainting, nausea or vomiting)	• If the wound is bleeding, apply direct pressure with a clean cloth or absorbent pad. • Wash the wound with clean, running tap water for about 5 minutes or until there appears to be no foreign matter in the wound. • Apply triple antibiotic lotion or cream to speed healing and reduce infection. • Cover the area with an adhesive bandage or gauze pad. • Change the dressing frequently. • **Do not** touch the white (sterile) side of the dressing. • **Do not** assume that a minor wound is clean.
Bruise[cos]	A bruise is caused by broken vessels leaking blood under the skin. • Pain • Swelling • Discoloration	• Apply ice to the injury to reduce pain, bleeding, and swelling. • To prevent cold injury, place a thin towel or cloth between the cold source and the skin. • Limit application to no more than 20 minutes.
Splinter	If a splinter is not removed, the wound may become inflamed and infected. Most splinters are removed easily at home or in the workplace.	• Using a pair of tweezers, grab the protruding end of the splinter and pull it out along the direction it entered. • If the splinter is under the skin or difficult to grab, use a needle or pin to uncover the splinter end. First sterilize the needle by soaking it in rubbing alcohol or placing the tip in a flame; wash your hands with soap. Then use the needle to gently remove the skin over the splinter. Use the tip of the needle to lift the end of the splinter out.[59] • If a splinter appears deeply embedded or you are able to remove only a piece of it, the wound should be seen by a health care professional.[24]

CAUTION!

Tetanus is a severe and often fatal infection associated with wounds. A tetanus shot is recommended if the victim does not know when his or her last tetanus vaccination was, or if it has been 10 years or longer since the last known vaccination.[25] A tetanus booster is recommended within 5 years for wounds with a high potential for infection, such as contaminated wounds, ragged wounds, and puncture wounds.

Have a wound evaluated by a health care professional when the wound has the following characteristics:

- Won't stop bleeding with firm direct pressure
- Is deep or longer than 1/2 inch, or about 1 centimeter (these may need closing with stitches or skin glue)
- Is on the face, especially when close to the eye
- Involves injury to underlying structures
- Was caused by a dirty or rusty object
- Has dirt, stones, or gravel stuck in it
- Was caused by an animal or human bite
- Is extremely painful
- Is infected (warm, red, swollen, or draining)

If you are concerned and have questions, you should not hesitate to contact your health care professional.

Burns

Burns have several causes:

- *Thermal burns* are caused by the sun, fire, hot liquids or objects, and hot gases.
- *Electrical burns* are caused by contact with electrical wires, current, or lightning.
- *Chemical burns* are caused by contact with wet or dry chemicals.

Burns on the face, hands, feet, and genitals can be particularly serious. Burns can inflict tremendous damage to the body. They can cause extreme pain, scarring, massive infection, organ failure, and death. **If a victim is on fire, tell him or her to stop, drop, and roll. If the victim is in contact with electricity, shut off the power.**

Special Concerns for Children and Older Adults

Minor burns in children are extremely common. Severe burns in children can result in prolonged suffering, disability, disfigurement, and impaired physical and mental development.[27] Age and chronic disease contribute to a higher frequency of complications and death in older adults who have burn injuries.

Take note of the following causes of burns to children:

- Hot-water scalds are twice as common as thermal burns in young children and typically occur when toddlers reach up and pull a pot of hot water off the stove and onto them.[28]
- Many fire-related injuries and deaths are caused by children under 5 years of age playing with matches or lighters, often in a bedroom. Keep matches and lighters in a secured drawer or cabinet.
- Use extra caution when working near energized power lines. Keep a safe distance between power lines and ladders, tools, and work materials.

	Signs and symptoms	First aid
Major[26] (third degree)	• Dry or leathery white or blackened, charred skin • Burns involving hands, face, eyes, ears, feet, and genitals • Electrical burns • Burns involving smoke inhalation, fractures, or other injury	**Assess, alert, and attend to the ABCs** • Expose the burn. • Cut and gently lift away any clothing covering the burned area. • If clothing is stuck to the burn, do not remove it. • If the victim is in contact with a liquid chemical, immediately flush the chemical with large amounts of water. • Remove jewelry, if possible (burns cause swelling). • Separate fingers or toes with dry, sterile, nonadhesive dressings. • Lightly cover the burn area with a dry, sterile bandage or a clean sheet if the burned area is large. • If it's available and you are properly trained, give emergency oxygen.
Minor[cos] (first or second degree)	• Pain • Redness • Swelling • Blisters	• Expose the burn. • Cool heat burns with cold water as quickly as possible and continue cooling at least until the pain is relieved. • After cooling, cover the burn with a dry, sterile bandage or a clean dressing. • Protect the burn from pressure and friction. • Immediate cooling of minor burns will reduce the swelling, infection, and depth of the injury. It will allow faster healing with less scarring. • Do not pop burn blisters. • Do not apply ointment, butter, ice, medications, cream, oil, spray, or any other substance to a burn.

CAUTION!

Consider any fallen or broken wire extremely dangerous. Do not touch (or allow your clothing to touch) a wire, victim, or vehicle that is possibly energized. Do not approach within 8 feet (2.4 meters) of it. Notify the local utility and have trained personnel sent to the scene. **Never** attempt to handle wires yourself unless you are properly trained and equipped. Once the power is off, assess, alert, and attend to the ABCs. The victim may need CPR and defibrillation (see chapters 3 and 4). Burns may be present at the points where the current entered and exited the body. All victims of electric shock require medical assessment because the extent of the injury may not be apparent.

Bites and Stings

Most bites and stings cause only minor swelling, redness, pain, and itching that last from a few hours to a few days. First aid is usually all that is needed to relieve the pain and itching of minor reactions. However, the bites and stings from venomous snakes, insects, or marine animals can cause intense pain and swelling. If not treated promptly and correctly, they can even cause serious illness or death. Bites from humans and other animals, such as dogs, cats, bats, raccoons, and rats, can cause severe injury and infection, including tetanus and rabies. Some people have severe allergic reactions to bites or stings that can be life threatening.

All wounds, including those caused by bites and stings, require the same general approach: Control bleeding, reduce pain, and prevent infection. Occasionally, the most important first aid measure is rapid transport to comprehensive medical care.[29] See the following table for specific recommendations.

	Signs and symptoms	First aid
Venomous snakebite (cottonmouth, rattlesnake)	• Single or double fang marks • Bleeding • Intense, burning pain and local swelling • If untreated, the swelling may involve the entire limb within hours • Whole-body effects include nausea, vomiting, sweating, fever, weakness, numbness, altered mental status, and shock	• If the site is bleeding, apply direct pressure with a clean cloth or absorbent pad. • Remove jewelry and constrictive clothing. • Cover the bite with an adhesive bandage or gauze pad. • Keep the injured part immobilized below heart level. • Keep the victim warm, reassured, and quiet. • Seek medical attention. • Do not cut through snakebite wounds or apply suctioning, ice, or tourniquets. These actions are of no proven value and may be dangerous.[30] **Severe reaction** Assess, alert, and attend to the ABCs.
Venomous snakebite (coral snake [cos])	• Pain and swelling may be minimal or absent. • Abdominal pain may occur (within hours of the bite). • Whole-body effects (may be delayed up to 6 hours) include nausea, vomiting, sweating, weakness, altered mental status, rapid heartbeat, drooling, difficulty breathing, stoppage of breathing.[31,32]	• Remove jewelry and constrictive clothing. • Apply a pressure bandage around the entire length of the bitten extremity to slow the spread of venom. The pressure bandage should be snug but not so tight that you cannot slip a finger under it. • Keep the injured part immobilized below heart level. • Keep the victim warm, reassured, and quiet. • Seek medical attention. **Severe reaction** Assess, alert, and attend to the ABCs.

Signs and symptoms	First aid
Venomous spider bite (widow, brown, or violin spiders)	• Bite site tender, swollen, painful, itchy, red • Puncture marks, bleeding • Heat over affected area • Whole-body effects include cramping pain and muscular rigidity in the abdomen or shoulders, back, and chest; fever; chills; rash; anxiety; weakness; nausea or vomiting; allergic reaction; difficulty breathing	• Remove jewelry and constrictive clothing. • Wash the site with clean, running tap water for several minutes. • Cover the area with an adhesive bandage or gauze pad. • Apply ice to the injury to reduce pain and swelling.[33-36] To prevent cold injury, place a thin towel or cloth between the cold source and the skin. Limit application to 20 minutes or less. • Keep the victim warm, reassured, and quiet. • Seek medical attention. **Severe reaction** Assess, alert, and attend to the ABCs.
Bees, wasps, fire ants	**Minor reaction** Bite site painful, red, swollen, itchy **Moderate reaction** Bite-site reaction expands slowly to more than 4 inches (10 centimeters) across **Severe reaction** Whole-body effects include • allergic reaction (can be fatal) • hives (raised itchy bumps on skin) • itching all over body • swelling of mouth or throat or both • shortness of breath or difficulty breathing • nausea or vomiting • chest pain or palpitations • anxiety or weakness • fainting	**Minor reaction** • If the stinger is present, remove it as quickly as possible. • Remove jewelry and constrictive clothing. • Wash the site with clean, running tap water for several minutes. • Cover the area with an adhesive bandage or gauze pad. • Apply ice to the injury to reduce pain and swelling. To prevent cold injury, place a thin towel or cloth between the cold source and the skin. Limit application to 20 minutes or less.[37] • Consider using over-the-counter anti-itch medications such as calamine lotion or Benadryl. **Moderate reaction** Seek medical attention. **Severe reaction** • Assess, alert, and attend to the ABCs. • If the victim has a history of hypersensitivity and carries a lifesaving epinephrine auto-injector prescribed by a physician, help him or her use it (see section titled Severe Allergic Reaction [Anaphylaxis] on page 35). If the victim is unable to use it, you should administer it.

(continued)

Signs and symptoms	First aid
Ticks	

	Signs and symptoms	First aid
Ticks	**Minor reaction** Bite site red, itchy, burning **Severe reaction** Whole-body effects (days to weeks after) include • fever or headache • confusion, anxiety, or weakness • fainting, nausea, or vomiting • difficulty breathing • chest pain or palpitations	**Minor reaction** • To remove a tick, grasp it close to the skin with tweezers (or use a commercially available tick removal tool). If tweezers or a tool is not available, use your fingers protected by gloves. Pull straight up with a steady, slow motion.[38, 39] • If the site bleeds, apply direct pressure with a clean cloth or absorbent pad. • Wash the site with clean, running tap water for about 5 minutes or until there appears to be no foreign matter in the wound. • Apply triple antibiotic lotion or cream. • Cover the area with an adhesive bandage or gauze pad. • Change the dressing frequently. • If portions of the tick remain embedded in the skin, or symptoms of severe reaction develop, seek medical attention. • **Do not** use fingernail polish, petroleum jelly, a glowing hot match, or alcohol to remove a tick. • **Do not** jerk, crush, squeeze, or puncture the tick. These actions are of no proven value and may cause additional injury.
Fire coral, sea anemones, jellyfish	**Minor reaction** Sting site painful, raised, red, itchy rash **Severe reaction** Whole-body effects include • shortness of breath or difficulty breathing • nausea or vomiting • anxiety, weakness, or fainting • chest pain or palpitations	**Minor reaction** • Carefully wipe off stingers or tentacles with a towel or remove with gloves. • Remove jewelry and constrictive clothing. Apply household vinegar to decrease symptoms.[40] • Consider using over-the-counter pain medications such as Tylenol and anti-itch medications such as calamine lotion or Benadryl. **Severe reaction** Assess, alert, and attend to the ABCs.

Signs and symptoms		First aid
Stingray sting	**Minor reaction** • Sting site very painful • Minor bleeding, swelling • Blue, then red tissue color **Severe reaction** Whole-body effects include • shortness of breath or difficulty breathing • headache • nausea or vomiting • anxiety, weakness, or fainting • chest pain or palpitations • muscle cramps, pain, or paralysis • seizure	**Minor reaction** • If the site is bleeding, apply direct pressure with a clean cloth or absorbent pad. • Remove jewelry and constrictive clothing. • Placing the injured area in water as hot as the victim can tolerate for 30 to 90 minutes can dramatically relieve pain.[41] • Seek medical attention. **Severe reaction** Assess, alert, and attend to the ABCs.
Human or animal	**Minor or moderate bite** • Bite, bruise, or break in skin Signs of infection • Increasing pain • Bite-site redness • Swelling, pus, warmth, red streaks, fever **Severe bite** • Large amount of blood pumping, gushing, or pouring from an open wound • Pain • Shock	**Minor or moderate bite** • If the site is bleeding, apply direct pressure with a clean cloth or absorbent pad. • Wash the site with clean, running tap water for about 5 minutes. • Cover the area with an adhesive bandage or gauze pad. • Apply ice to the injury to reduce pain, bleeding, and swelling. To prevent cold injury, place a thin towel or cloth between the cold source and skin. Limit application to 20 minutes or less. • Seek medical attention. **Severe bite** • Assess, alert, and attend to the ABCs. • Control severe bleeding and care for shock. • Save any tissue parts that were bitten off. Treat them as you would an amputation.

Special Concerns for Children and Older Adults

Dogs bite millions of people every year, causing serious injuries and even death. Children who are younger than 10 years of age represent the high-risk group for dog attacks. The majority of the dogs who attack children are familiar to them.[42] Teach children basic safety around dogs and review it regularly.

Aging can make an older person more vulnerable to the beginnings of infection. Always watch any bite, sting, or break in the skin for signs of infection, especially in older adults.

Prevention

To prevent bites and stings, do the following:

• Respect and use caution around insects and animals. Do not harass them.

• Wear an effective insect repellent when outside.

• Shuffle your feet while walking or wading through water to scare stingrays away.

Dental Injuries

Because they help determine facial appearance and function, traumatic injuries to the mouth, teeth, and jaw can have significant physical and emotional effects. Injuries involving the mouth and teeth often result from falls, sport-related injuries, fighting, car crashes, and running into stationary objects. Teeth can be dislocated, broken, or knocked out (avulsed). A permanent tooth that is knocked out can be put back in.

	First aid
Dislocated or broken tooth	• If the lips, teeth, or gums are bleeding, apply direct pressure with a clean cloth or absorbent pad (or have the victim gently bite down on an absorbent pad). • Arrange for the victim to be seen by a dentist immediately.

Knocked-out tooth	• If the lips, teeth, or gums are bleeding, apply direct pressure with a clean cloth or absorbent pad (or have the victim do it).
	• Handle the tooth only by the chewing surface (crown).
	• Place the knocked-out tooth in one of the following solutions:
	  - Save-A-Tooth emergency tooth preserving system, a scientifically designed, FDA-approved system of preserving knocked-out teeth for up to 24 hours.[43]
	  - Fresh whole milk, which can preserve cells for up to 6 hours.[44]
	  - Cold low-fat milk, contact lens solution, or Gatorade, which can serve as an alternative to fresh whole milk for up to an hour.[45, 46]
	• **Do not** put an avulsed tooth in water! Water is harmful to tooth cells.
	• Get to the dentist as quickly as possible. The faster you act, the better your chances of saving the tooth. Thirty minutes or less gives the best chance for success.
	• **Do not** touch the root of the tooth (the part of the tooth usually in the gum).
	• **Do not** scrub an avulsed tooth or remove any attached tissue fragments.
	• **Do not** allow an avulsed tooth to dry.
	• **Do not** wrap an avulsed tooth in tissues, cloth, or gauze.

Eye Injuries

Eye injuries range from minor irritation to very severe injury. Severe eye injuries are frequently caused by objects in the eye, burns, and blunt injuries. Any of these conditions can lead to a permanent loss of vision.[47] The following are signs and symptoms of eye injuries:

- Pain, redness, stinging, burning, itching
- Bleeding, bruising, or black eye
- Something stuck in the eye
- Sensitivity to light
- Decreased or double vision
- Problem with or loss of vision
- Anxiety, pale or clammy skin, weakness or fainting, nausea or vomiting

Special Concerns for Children and Older Adults

Do not allow children to rub their eyes. All children with eye injuries should be evaluated, especially if they complain of any visual problems, scratching sensations, or pain.

The risk of eye injury declines with age. Most eye injuries are due to falls.[48] If the victim is responsive, in addition to caring for the eye injury, check the victim for hidden injuries that may have occurred because of the fall (i.e., do a physical assessment).

Prevention

Tradespeople (machinists, welders, metalworkers) have three to four times more occupational eye injuries than the overall population. Males aged 17 to 24 are at the greatest risk. The consistent use of eye protection during hazardous activities—at home and at work—could prevent many eye injuries.[49]

	First aid
Minor irritated eye	• Rinse the affected eye with a saline solution. • Tap water may be used if no saline solution is available. Use a drinking fountain, faucet, or garden hose running slowly. • If the victim continues to have pain or feels that something is still in the eye, or if the object cannot be removed, cover the eye lightly with a gauze pad or a clean cloth and seek medical attention.
Object stuck in eye	Protect the eye from further injury: • Tape the bottom half of a foam or paper cup over the victim's eye to help keep both the eye and the object from moving. • Lightly cover the uninjured eye with gauze or a clean cloth. Because the eyes move together, covering both helps keep the injured eye and object from moving and causing further injury. • Since the victim has both eyes covered, you must become the eyes of the victim. Protect the victim from further harm. Keep the victim quiet and safe and reassure him or her with a calm, compassionate, and confident tone of voice. • Seek immediate medical care. • **Do not** try to remove the object. • **Do not** allow the victim to rub or to apply pressure to the injured eye. Pressure can damage the delicate fibers of the optic nerve, which connects the eye with the brain.
Chemical burn[cos]	• Immediately flood the eye with a large amount of water. Use a drinking fountain, faucet, or garden hose. • After you have finished washing the eye, seek immediate medical care. • **Do not** place a cup over the eye. • **Do not** bandage the eye.

Nosebleeds

Most nosebleeds are not serious and can be handled easily, but in rare cases, a nosebleed can lead to massive bleeding and even death. Nosebleeds affect people of all ages but are most common in younger children and older adults. Applying ice to the victim's neck is not effective in controlling a nosebleed.[50]

Signs and symptoms	First aid
• Bleeding from one nostril • Blood can drip down the throat or into the stomach, causing a victim to spit or vomit blood • Anxiety, pale or clammy skin, weakness, fainting, nausea or vomiting	• Have the victim sit up straight with the head tilted forward. • Pinch the nose with thumb and index finger for 10 minutes. • Have the victim spit out any blood that collects in the mouth. • If the bleeding does not stop, seek immediate medical care. • **Do not** tilt the victim's head back or have the victim lie down. These actions may cause the victim to swallow blood and vomit. • **Do not** pack gauze in the nose.

Limb, Spine, and Head Injuries

As a first aid provider, you might need to treat injuries to the arms and legs at some time. More serious are spine and head injuries that can lead to permanent damage and loss of function.

Injuries to Limbs[COS]

Bones, joints, and muscles give the body shape, allow movement, and protect vital internal organs. Injuries to the bones, joints, and muscles of the limbs are common injuries that may be cared for by a first aid provider. Prompt recognition and first aid for limb injuries are important in reducing pain, preventing further injury, and decreasing permanent damage (see table on page 55 and Skill Guide 5 on page 57). **If a painful, deformed, or swollen limb is blue or extremely pale, activate EMS or your emergency action plan immediately.**

Splinting is the most common procedure for limiting limb movement. Figure 2.10 shows how to immobilize an injured arm, and figure 2.11 shows how you might improvise a leg splint. Apply a splint only in these conditions:

- EMS personnel are delayed or not available (e.g., during a natural disaster or a terrorist attack).

- You can do so without causing further injury or pain.

Before beginning, gather whatever splinting materials are available. If possible, use at least four ties (two above and two below the fracture) to secure the splints. You can use a variety of materials to improvise a splint:

- **Soft:** Towels, blankets, or pillows tied with bandaging materials or soft cloths

- **Rigid:** Cardboard, wood, a folded magazine, a backpacker's sleeping pad

Follow these guidelines when you splint a limb:

- Immobilize the limb above and below the injury.

- Splint it in the position in which it was found.

- Pad the splints where they touch any bony part of the body to help prevent circulation problems.

- After splinting, check the limb frequently for swelling, paleness, or numbness. If present, loosen the splint.

Signs and symptoms		First aid
Closed fracture, strain, sprain, dislocation: no open wound Open fracture: open wound. May have bone sticking out.	**Closed** • Sharp pain • Swelling • Deformity • Tenderness • Bruising • Joint locked into position • Anxiety, pale or clammy skin, weakness, fainting **Open** • Bleeding • Pain • Swelling • Deformity • Anxiety, pale or clammy skin, weakness, fainting, nausea or vomiting • Substantial blood loss from open fractures is possible[51]	**For open or closed injury:** • If necessary, expose the injury by gently cutting away clothing. • If a bone is sticking out of the body, control bleeding by applying gentle pressure around it. • Cover open wounds with a sterile or clean dressing. • Remove all jewelry from the injured part and give it to the victim (injuries cause swelling). • **Do not** remove shoes or boots unless there is severe bleeding from the foot. • Apply ice to the injury to reduce pain, bleeding, and swelling. • Improper use of ice packs or other frozen material can cause a severe frostbite injury.[52] To prevent cold injury, place a thin towel or cloth between the cold source and the skin. Limit application to 20 minutes or less. • Gently place your hands above and below the injury site to limit movement and prevent further injury. • Comfort, calm, and reassure the victim. • **Do not** straighten a painful, swollen, or deformed arm or leg. • **Do not** push a bone back under the skin. • **Do not** allow the victim to put weight on a leg, ankle, or foot injury.

CAUTION!

Sharp broken bone ends can cut tissue, muscle, blood vessels, and nerves when moved. Assume all painful, swollen, or deformed injuries to a limb include broken bone ends.

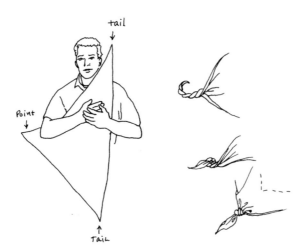

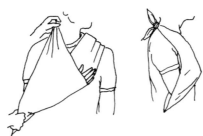

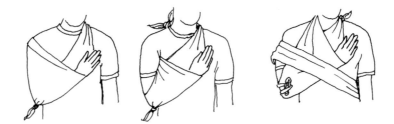

Figure 2.10 Sling and swath for injured arm.

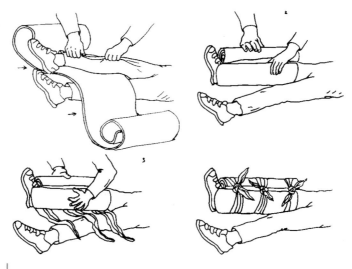

Figure 2.11 Improvised leg splint.

Injured Limb

Emergency Action Steps

1. **Assess scene.** If the scene is unsafe or at any time becomes unsafe, **get out!**
2. **Assess victim.** Is the victim responsive? Identify yourself; ask if it's OK to help. If the victim appears to be weak, seriously ill, or injured, follow steps 3 and 4.
3. **Alert.** Call EMS (9-1-1) or activate your emergency action plan.
4. **Attend to the ABCs.** Ensure an open airway and normal breathing, then control bleeding and manage shock.

Cover Open Wounds

- Use a sterile dressing.
- If a bone is sticking out of the body, control bleeding by applying gentle pressure around it.

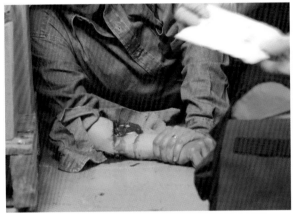

Apply Ice or Cold Pack

- This will decrease pain, bleeding, and swelling.
- Limit application to 20 minutes or less.

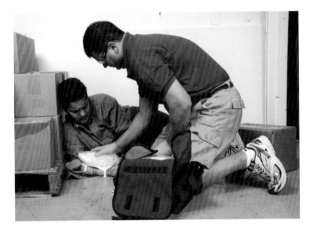

Manually Stabilize Injured Limb

- Gently place your hands above and below the injury to limit movement and to prevent further injury while awaiting EMS.

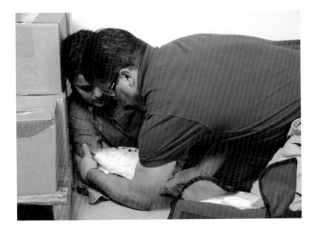

Injuries to the Spine

Injuries to the spine[cos] cause damage to the bones of the spine, the spinal cord, or the tissues and blood vessels surrounding the spinal cord. Spinal cord injury causes great physical and emotional stress. The primary goal of first aid is to prevent further injury (see Skill Guide 6). **If an unresponsive victim is lying flat on his or her back and has debris, blood, or secretions in the mouth that causes difficult breathing or you must leave to get help, use the HAINES position to protect the airway.**

Special Concerns for Children and Older Adults

Spinal injury in children is rare, but the risk is greatest when the child has multiple injuries or chest injuries.[53] Distress and discomfort may make it difficult to restrict spinal motion in a child. Do your best to hold the child's head in the position in which it was found.

Loss of normal bone density, mass, and strength make older people more likely to fracture bones, including spinal bones. Older adults who have other medical problems that make them prone to falling (for example, stroke) may also be more vulnerable to spinal injury. Do your best to manually restrict the victim's head in the position in which it was found.

Signs and symptoms	First aid
<ul><li>Altered mental status</li><li>Obvious injury to the neck, head, or back</li><li>Numbness, tingling, burning, or loss of sensation in the hands, fingers, feet, or toes</li><li>Spinal pain, pressure, or tenderness</li><li>Multiple injuries, including open or closed fractures</li><li>Weakness or paralysis in any part of the body</li><li>Loss of bladder or bowel control</li><li>Bullet or stab wound to the head, neck, or chest</li><li>A headfirst dive into shallow water</li></ul> **Assume a spinal injury has occurred when the victim has the following conditions:** <ul><li>Has been exposed to physical force and has any of the signs and symptoms listed previously.</li><li>Was in a motor vehicle (car, truck, motorcycle, ATV) or bicycle crash (occupant or pedestrian).</li><li>Fell from greater than a standing height.</li><li>Has been exposed to physical force and appears drunk or older than 65.</li></ul>	**Tell a responsive victim not to move.** <ul><li>Place your hands on both sides of the victim's head to stabilize it.</li><li>Keep the head, neck, and spine in line.</li><li>Comfort, calm, and reassure the victim.</li><li>**Do not** ask the injured victim to move in order to try to find a pain response.</li><li>**Do not** move the injured victim to test for a pain response.</li><li>**Do not** move the injured victim to perform a physical assessment.</li><li>**Do not** bend, twist, or lift the injured victim's head or body.</li><li>**Do not** move the injured victim before medical help arrives unless his or her life is in danger.</li><li>**Do not** remove a helmet if a spinal injury is suspected.</li></ul>

CAUTION!

Pain and loss of function usually accompany a spinal injury, but the absence of pain does not mean that the victim has not been significantly injured. If you suspect a victim could possibly have a spinal injury, assume one is present!

Suspected Spinal Injury

Emergency Action Steps

1. **Assess scene.** If the scene is unsafe or at any time becomes unsafe, **get out!**
2. **Assess victim.** Is the victim responsive? Identify yourself; ask if it's OK to help. If the victim appears to be weak, seriously ill, or injured, follow steps 3 and 4.
3. **Alert.** Call EMS (9-1-1) or activate your emergency action plan.
4. **Attend to the ABCs.** Ensure an open airway and normal breathing, then control bleeding.

Manually Stabilize Suspected Spinal Injury

- Tell the responsive victim not to move.
- Place your hands on both sides of the victim's head to stabilize it.
- Keep the victim's head, neck, and spine in line.
- Comfort, calm, and reassure the victim.

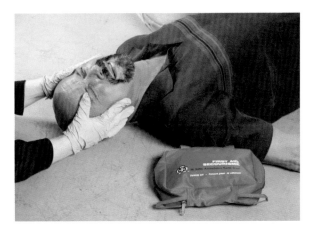

Protect the Airway

- If the victim is or becomes unresponsive and has debris or blood in the mouth or has difficulty breathing from secretions in the mouth, or you must leave to get help, use the HAINES position to protect the airway (see Skill Guide 3 on page 30 for this procedure).

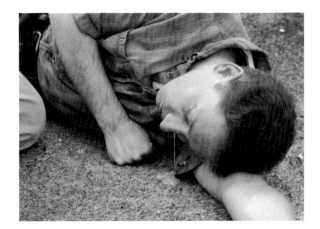

Injuries to the Brain and Skull

Injuries to the brain and skull[cos] can be closed or open. A typical closed injury is a concussion, in which the brain is bruised from impact against the inside of the skull. An open injury, such as that caused by a bullet, can cause long-lasting functional impairment or death.

Injuries to the brain and skull are a worldwide problem. In the United States, firearms top injuries from motor vehicle crashes as the largest single cause of death associated with brain injury.[54,55]

Special Concerns for Children and Older Adults

If a child begins to play or run immediately after getting a bump on the head, serious injury is unlikely. However, the child should be seen by a health care professional and closely watched for 24 hours after the incident. You should contact the child's doctor if the child vomits more than once. Vomiting is more common in younger children and is less likely to be an urgent sign of danger than it is in an adult.[56]

Injuries to the brain and skull caused by falling are highest among people 65 years of age and older. First aid for older adults with an injury to the skull or brain is the same as for any victim.

Prevention

Here are some prevention tips:

- Practices that have been associated with reducing firearm injuries in homes with children and guns include keeping the gun locked and unloaded and storing ammunition locked in a separate location.[57]

- Helmets reduce biking-related head and facial injuries for people of all ages in all types of accidents, including those involving motor vehicles.[58]

- Always use safety equipment during activities that could result in head injury. These include seat belts, bicycle or motorcycle helmets, and hard hats.

Signs and symptoms	First aid
- Unresponsiveness - Confusion or sleepiness - Clear or bloody fluid draining from the nose, mouth, or ears - External bleeding or protruding brain matter - Facial bruising, swelling, or scalp wound - Nausea or vomiting - Seizures - Severe headache or stiff neck - Inability to move one or more limbs - Changes in pupil size or shape - Inability to hear, see, taste, or smell - Abnormal behavior	**Assess, alert, and attend the ABCs** - If the wound is bleeding, place an absorbent pad directly over the area. If the pad becomes soaked with blood, apply another one over it. Do not remove blood-soaked dressings. - If you suspect a spinal injury, manually stabilize the victim's head and neck. - **Do not** move the victim unless it is necessary. - **Do not** wash a head wound that is deep or has major bleeding. - **Do not** remove any object sticking out of a wound. - **Do not** remove a helmet if you suspect a serious head injury. - **Do not** pick up a child if you suspect a head, neck, or back injury. **Seizures or convulsions** - Involuntary jerking may occur after a brain or skull injury. - Protect the victim from hitting nearby objects. - **Do not** try to stop the jerking movements in a seizure. Doing so can cause injury to the bones, joints, muscles, and soft tissue. - **Do not** place an object in a seizure victim's mouth. Doing so is dangerous and may cause further injury.

References

1. NFASAB. Definition of first aid. *Circulation* 2005; 112:IV-196-IV-203. American Heart Association and the American National Red Cross.

2. Shenefelt, R. Emotional aspects of basic life support. Presentation. Scientific Program of the New Zealand Resuscitation Council Conference, Wellington, NZ 1999 November.

3. U.S. Department of Veterans Affairs. Types of debriefing following disasters. www.ncptsd. va.gov/facts/disasters/fs_type_debriefings_ disaster.html. Accessed 2006 March 17.

4. U.S. Department of Veterans Affairs. Brief tips about self-care and self-help following disasters. www.ncptsd.va.gov/facts/disasters/fs_self_care_ brief.html. Accessed 19 March 2006.

5. Aehlert, B. *Pediatric advanced life support.* Study guide, chapter 2: Patient assessment. St. Louis: Mosby; 2005.

6. Rathgeber J, et al. Influence of different types of recovery positions on perfusion indices of the forearm. *Resuscitation* 1996 July; 32(1):13-7.

7. Gunn BD, et al. How should an unconscious person with a suspected neck injury be positioned? *Prehospital Disaster Med* 1995 October-December; 10(4):239-44.

8. Blake WE, Stillman BC, Eizenberg N, Briggs C, McMeeken JM. The position of the spine in the recovery position: An experimental comparison between the lateral recovery position and the modified HAINES position. *Resuscitation* 2002 June; 53(3):289-97.

9. Adapted from Community Emergency Response Team (CERT) Program. Participant Manual, Unit 3: Disaster medical operations—part 1. www.citizencorps.gov/cert/training_mat. shtm#CERTSM. Accessed 2006 August 30.

10. American Academy of Pediatrics, American Public Health Association, National Resource Center for Health and Safety in Child Care. 2002. Caring for our children. National Health and Safety Performance Standards: Guidelines for Out-of-Home Child Care Programs. 2nd ed. http://nrc.uchsc.edu/CFOC/XMLVersion/ NewTOCwoSubs.xml. Accessed 2006 August.

11. Asthma and Allergy Foundation of America. Student asthma action card. http://aafa.org/index. cfm. Accessed 2006 August.

12. Meridian Medical Technologies. EpiPen and EpiPen Jr. Patient insert. www.epipen.com/ default.aspx. Accessed 2006 August.

13. Pediatrics Committee, National Association of EMS Physicians. Anaphylactic shock treated with auto-injector device. EMSC Partnership for Children/National Association of EMS physicians model pediatric protocols: 2003 revision. *Prehosp Emer Care* 2004 October-December; 8(4):359.

14. Diabetes. www.emedicinehealth.com/insulin_ reaction/article_em.htm. Accessed 2006 August 30.

15. U.S. Department of Labor, Occupational Safety & Health Administration. Regulations (standards—29 CFR) respiratory protection 1910.134. www.osha.gov/pls/oshaweb/owadisp.show_ document?p_table=STANDARDS&p_id=12716. Accessed 2006 August 30.

16. Watson W, et al. 2003 annual report of the American Association of Poison Control Centers. Toxic exposure surveillance system. *American Journal of Emergency Medicine* 2004 September; 22(5).

17. Bergeron MF. Heat cramps: Fluid and electrolyte challenges during tennis in the heat. *J Sci Med Sport* March 2003; 6(1):19-27.

18. Hoppe J, Sinert R, Kunihiro A, Foster J. March 16, 2006. Heat exhaustion and heatstroke. www. emedicine.com/emerg/topic236.htm. Accessed 2006 August.

19. Semenza JC, Rubin CH, Falter KH, Selanikio JD, Flanders WD, Howe HL, Wilhelm JL. Heat-related deaths during the July 1995 heat wave in Chicago. *N Engl J Med* 1996 July; 11;335(2):84-90.

20. Rajpal RC, Weisskopf MG, Rumm PD, Peterson PL, Jentzen JM, Blair K, Foldy S. Wisconsin, July 1999 heat wave: An epidemiologic assessment. *Wisconsin Medical Journal* 2000 August; 99(5):41-4.

21. Guard A, Gallagher SS. Heat related deaths to young children in parked cars: An analysis of 171 fatalities in the United States, 1995-2002. *Inj Prev* 2005 February; 11(1):33-7.

22. Long WB III, Edlich RF, Winters KL, Britt LD. Cold injuries. *Long Term Eff Med Implants* 2005; 15(1):67-78.

23. Perez E, National Library of Medicine. Frostbite. March 21, 2006. www.nlm.nih.gov/medlineplus/ency/article/000057.htm. Accessed 2006 August.

24. EMedicineHealth. Splinters. August 10, 2005. www.emedicinehealth.com/articles/20266-6.asp. Accessed 2006 August.

25. Pascual FB, McGinley EL, Zanardi LR, Cortese MM, Murphy TV. Tetanus surveillance—United States, 1998-2000. *MMWR Surveill Summ* 2003 June 20; 52(3):1-8.

26. Demling RH, DeSanti L. Initial management of the burn patient. www.burnsurgery.org/Modules/initial_mgmt/index_initial_mgmt.htm Accessed 2006 August.

27. Peleg K, Goldman S, Sikron F. January 21, 2005. Burn prevention programs for children: Do they reduce burn-related hospitalizations? *Burns* 2005 May; 31(3):347-50.

28. Drago DA. Kitchen scalds and thermal burns in children five years and younger. *Pediatrics* 2005 January; 115(1):10-6.

29. Merck Manual of Diagnosis and Therapy Section 23. Poisoning, chapter 308: Bites and stings. www.merck.com/mrkshared/mmanual/home.jsp. Accessed 2006 August.

30. Pochanugool C, et al. Venomous snakebite in Thailand II: Clinical experience. *Mil Med* 1998 May; 163(5):318-23.

31. Kularatne SA. Common krait (*Bungarus caeruleus*) bite in Anuradhapura, Sri Lanka: A prospective clinical study, 1996-98. *Postgrad Med J* 2002 May; 78(919):276-80.

32. Hughes A. Observation of snakebite victims: Is twelve hours still necessary? *Emerg Med (Fremantle)* 2003 October-December; 15(5-6):511-7.

33. Wilson DC, King LE Jr. Spiders and spider bites. *Dermatol Clin* 1990 April; 8(2):277-86.

34. Sams HH, Hearth SB, Long LL, Wilson DC, Sanders DH, King LE Jr. Nineteen documented cases of Loxosceles reclusa envenomation. *J Am Acad Dermatol* 2001 April; 44(4):603-8.

35. Leach J, Bassichis B, Itani K. Brown recluse spider bites to the head: Three cases and a review. *Ear Nose Throat J* 2004 July; 83(7):465-70.

36. National Library of Medicine. August 11, 2006. Black widow spider. www.nlm.nih.gov/medlineplus/ency/article/002858.htm. Accessed 2006 August.

37. Perez, E, National Library of Medicine. February 13, 2006. Fire ant. www.nlm.nih.gov/medlineplus/ency/article/002843.htm. Accessed 2006 August.

38. Stewart RL, Burgdorfer W, Needham GR. Evaluation of three commercial tick removal tools. *Wilderness Environ Med* 1998 Fall; 9(3):137-42.

39. Needham GR. Evaluation of five popular methods for tick removal. *Pediatrics* 1985 June; 75(6):997-1002.

40. EMedicine.com. August 10, 2005. Jellyfish stings. www.emedicinehealth.com/articles/6277-6.asp. Accessed 2006 August.

41. EMedicine.com. Stingray injury. August 10, 2005. www.emedicinehealth.com/articles/10751-6.asp. Accessed 2006 August.

42. Schalamon J, et al. Analysis of dog bites in children who are younger than 17 years. *Pediatrics* 2006 March; 117(3):e374-9.

43. U.S. Food and Drug Administration Center for Devices and Radiological Health. Device listing database. www.accessdata.fda.gov/scripts/cdrh/cfdocs/search/search.cfm?db=LST&ID=75054. Accessed 2006 August.

44. Hiltz J, Trope M. Vitality of human lip fibroblasts in milk, Hanks balanced salt solution and Viaspan storage media. *Endod Dent Traumatol* 1991 April; 7(2):69-72.

45. Harkacz OM Sr., Carnes DL Jr., Walker WA III. Determination of periodontal ligament cell viability in the oral rehydration fluid Gatorade and milks of varying fat content. *J Endod* 1997 November; 23(11):687-90.

46. Pileggi R, Dumsha TC, Nor JE. Assessment of post-traumatic PDL cells viability by a novel collagenase assay. *Dent Traumatol* 2002 August; 18(4):186-9.

47. Douglas RS, National Library of Medicine. April 8, 2005. Eye emergencies. www.nlm.nih.gov/medlineplus/ency/article/000054.htm. Accessed 2006 August.

48. EMedicineHealth.com. Angle recession glaucoma 2003-2005. www.emedicinehealth.com/articles/41766-1.asp. Accessed 2006 August.

49. Andreotti G, Lange JL, Brundage JF. The nature, incidence, and impact of eye injuries among US military personnel: implications for prevention. *Arch Ophthalmol* 2001 November; 119(11):1693-7.

50. Teymoortash A, Sesterhenn A, Kress R, Sapund-zhiev N, Werner JA. Efficacy of ice packs in the management of epistaxis. *Clin Otolaryngol Allied Sci* 2003 December; 28(6):545-7.

51. Pryor JP, Reilly PM. Initial care of the patient with blunt polytrauma. *Clin Orthop Relat Res* 2004 May; (422):30-6.

52. Graham CA, Stevenson J. Frozen chips: An unusual cause of severe frostbite injury. *Br J Sports Med* 2000 October; 34(5):382-3.

53. Martin BW, Dykes E, Lecky FE. Patterns and risks in spinal trauma. *Arch Dis Child* 2004 September; 89(9):860-5.

54. Adekoya N, Thurman DJ, White DD, Webb KW. Surveillance for traumatic brain injury deaths: United States, 1989-1998. *MMWR Surveill Summ* 2002 December 6; 51(10):1-14.

55. Langlois JA, et al. Traumatic brain injury-related hospital discharges: Results from a 14-state sur-veillance system, 1997. *MMWR Surveill Summ* 2003 June 27; 52(4):1-20.

56. U.S. Department of Health and Human Services, Centers for Disease Control and Prevention. October 8, 2004. Facts about concussion and brain injury. www.cdc.gov/ncipc/tbi/Section01. htm. Accessed 2006 August.

57. Grossman DC, et al. Gun storage practices and risk of youth suicide and unintentional firearm injuries. *JAMA* 2005 February 9; 293(6):707-14.

58. Thompson DC, Rivara FP, Thompson R. Helmets for preventing head and facial injuries in bicy-clists. Cochrane Database of Systematic Reviews 1999, Issue 4.

59. National Library of Medicine and National Institutes of Health. August 11, 2006. Splinter removal. www.nlm.nih.gov/medlineplus/ency/ article/002137.htm. Accessed 2006 August.

CPR and AED for the Community and Workplace

3

Note to readers: The procedures described in this chapter are intended **only** for community members and people who do not work in the health care field but who are required or just desire to have CPR and AED knowledge and skills on a volunteer basis. This includes emergency response teams in business, industry, and government; school bus drivers; adult residential care personnel; child care workers; teachers; parents; and babysitters. If you need to learn CPR on a professional basis (e.g., a professional rescuer, lifeguard, medical professional), you should read chapter 4. American Safety & Health Institute (ASHI) certification may be issued only when an ASHI-authorized instructor verifies that you have successfully completed and competently performed the required core knowledge and skill objectives of the program. By itself, this chapter does not constitute complete training.

In this book, the term *basic life support* (BLS) means recognizing signs of sudden cardiac arrest (SCA), heart attack, stroke, and foreign-body airway obstruction (FBAO); administering cardiopulmonary resuscitation (CPR); and using an automated external defibrillator (AED).[1]

The basic life support procedures and skills you will learn in this chapter include the following:

- How the respiratory and circulatory systems work
- How to identify types of heart disease and stroke and give first aid for them

- How to follow the emergency action steps for adults, children, and infants:
  - Rescue breathing
  - Chest compressions
  - Using an AED
- How to aid adults, children, and infants who are choking
- Key psychological and legal aspects of providing basic life support
- How to alter the standard emergency action steps to accommodate special conditions

Figure 3.1 shows the basic life support procedures to be taught in this chapter.

Universal Basic Life Support Procedures*

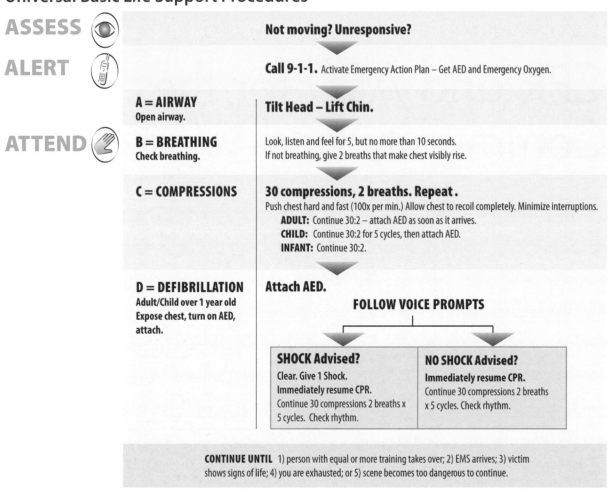

ASSESS — Not moving? Unresponsive?

ALERT — **Call 9-1-1.** Activate Emergency Action Plan – Get AED and Emergency Oxygen.

ATTEND

A = AIRWAY
Open airway.

Tilt Head – Lift Chin.

B = BREATHING
Check breathing.

Look, listen and feel for 5, but no more than 10 seconds.
If not breathing, give 2 breaths that make chest visibly rise.

C = COMPRESSIONS

30 compressions, 2 breaths. Repeat.
Push chest hard and fast (100x per min.) Allow chest to recoil completely. Minimize interruptions.
ADULT: Continue 30:2 – attach AED as soon as it arrives.
CHILD: Continue 30:2 for 5 cycles, then attach AED.
INFANT: Continue 30:2.

D = DEFIBRILLATION
Adult/Child over 1 year old
Expose chest, turn on AED,
attach.

Attach AED.
FOLLOW VOICE PROMPTS

SHOCK Advised?
Clear. Give 1 Shock.
Immediately resume CPR.
Continue 30 compressions 2 breaths x
5 cycles. Check rhythm.

NO SHOCK Advised?
Immediately resume CPR.
Continue 30 compressions 2 breaths
x 5 cycles. Check rhythm.

CONTINUE UNTIL 1) person with equal or more training takes over; 2) EMS arrives; 3) victim
shows signs of life; 4) you are exhausted; or 5) scene becomes too dangerous to continue.

Procedure adapted from *Circulation* 2005; 112: III-3, IV-21, IV-158 © 2005 International Liaison Committee on Resuscitation,
American Heart Association,® Inc. and European Resuscitation Council.

Figure 3.1   Universal basic life support procedures.

Respiratory System

When you provide BLS, you help the victim's respiratory and circulatory systems to function. Each cell of the body requires a regular supply of oxygen in order to stay alive. Because the body cannot store oxygen as it does food and water, we must continually breathe oxygen into the lungs. Respiration is the process of taking in oxygen and giving off carbon dioxide. The respiratory system is a collection of organs involved in this process. The system, shown in figure 3.2, is made up of *(a)* the lungs, *(b)* bronchial tubes, *(c)* nose, *(d)* mouth, *(e)* windpipe, and *(f)* diaphragm. When you take a breath, the diaphragm

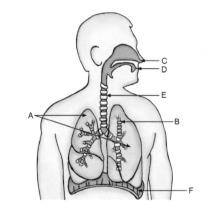

Figure 3.2   The respiratory system.

moves down and the chest moves out, drawing air into the lungs. This is called *inhalation.* The air we inhale contains approximately 21% oxygen. In the lungs, oxygen is absorbed into the bloodstream and circulated throughout the body. When the diaphragm moves up, air exits the lungs in *exhalation.* Carbon dioxide is released in the exhaled air. Not all of the oxygen is used by the body in the breathing process. Exhaled air contains about 16 to 17% oxygen. When this air is delivered during rescue breathing, there is still enough oxygen to support life.

Circulatory System

The circulatory system uses the bloodstream to deliver oxygen and nutrients to the body tissues and removes waste products from them. Figure 3.3 is a simplified drawing of the circulatory system. The driving force of the system is the heart *(a).* Special tissue runs throughout the heart that is capable of creating and conducting electric current. This electric current triggers the rhythmic mechanical contractions that create the flow of blood through the body's blood vessels and heart, which is known as circulation. Large vessels called arteries *(b)* carry oxygenated blood from the heart to body tissues. Capillaries *(c)* are where oxygen, nutrients, and waste products are exchanged and where arteries connect to veins *(d)* to return used blood back to the heart. From there, the used blood is sent to the lungs, where carbon dioxide is released and fresh oxygen is picked up. The fresh blood is returned to the heart, and the cycle repeats.

The body cannot survive when circulation stops. Brain tissue is especially sensitive to a lack of oxygen. External chest compressions combined with rescue breathing (CPR) are essential for providing blood flow to vital organs during cardiac arrest. Immediate CPR can double or triple a victim's chance of survival. Unfortunately, the majority of cardiac arrest survivors remain in a coma for varying lengths of time, and full brain recovery is rare.[2]

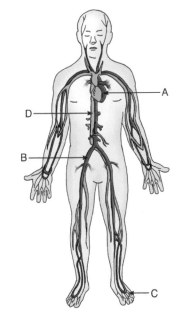

Figure 3.3   The circulatory system.

Universal Precautions

As described in chapter 1, universal precautions are a way to limit the spread of disease by preventing rescuers from having contact with blood and body fluids. To observe universal precautions means that whether or not you think the victim's blood or body fluid is infected, you act as if it is.

The risk of contracting a disease while giving BLS is extremely low. No documented cases exist of human immunodeficiency virus (HIV), hepatitis B (HBV), or hepatitis C (HCV) infection transmitted by mouth-to-mouth ventilation. The estimated risk for acquiring HIV, HBV, or HCV infection during basic life support is extremely low—about one in one million. There have been no reports of infection acquired during CPR training. Simple infection-control measures, including use of barrier devices, can reduce the risk for acquisition of an infectious disease during CPR and CPR training.[3]

While the risk of disease is low when you perform CPR, observing universal precautions with victims of all ages will make it lower. Using masks and wearing face shields allows you to perform rescue breathing without compromising your own health. These devices are usually available for all ages and sizes. They come with a replaceable one-way valve or filters to block contaminated fluids. All first aid kits should have at least one rescue breathing mask or face shield (see figure 3.4).

Be sure to wear other types of personal protective equipment as necessary, such as gloves and goggles. Follow the procedures that you learned in chapter 1 for preventing infection from pathogens.

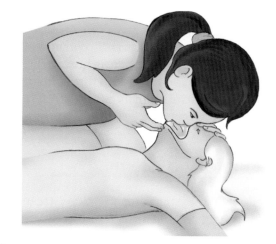

Figure 3.4 Rescue breathing with a face shield.

Heart Disease and Stroke

Heart disease and stroke—the main components of cardiovascular disease—are the leading causes of death for both men and women in the United States and account for nearly 40% of all deaths.[4] More than 927,000 Americans die of cardiovascular disease each year, which amounts to 1 death every 34 seconds. Heart disease and stroke are also leading causes of death in Canada.[5] By 2020 heart disease and stroke will become the leading cause of both death and disability worldwide; the number of deaths is projected to increase to more than 20 million a year.[6]

The major independent risk factors for heart disease and stroke are high blood pressure and high blood cholesterol. A 12- to 13-point reduction in blood pressure can reduce heart attacks by 21%, strokes by 37%, and all deaths from cardiovascular disease by 25%.[7]

Everyone should know the signs and symptoms of heart attack and stroke and the importance of calling 9-1-1 quickly; almost half (47%) of heart attack victims and about the same percentage of stroke victims die before EMS personnel arrive.[8] Family members of people who have had a recent heart attack should take CPR training and be familiar with the use of an automated external defibrillator (AED, described on page 71). Employers should consider the use of AEDs at their worksites to reduce the time to defibrillation with the goal of improving survival.[9] All designated responders who respond to victims with chest pain and suspected cardiac arrest should be trained to use an AED.

The next sections cover the signs and symptoms and first aid treatments for acute coronary syndrome, stroke (brain attack), and sudden cardiac arrest.

Lowering Your Risk for Cardiovascular Disease

You can lower your risk for cardiovascular disease by making healthy lifestyle choices such as these:

- Eat a healthy diet to prevent or reduce high blood pressure and high blood cholesterol. A healthy diet is high in fruits and vegetables, whole grains, and lean protein and low in saturated fat, cholesterol, trans fat, artificial preservatives, refined carbohydrate, and sugar.
- Maintain a healthy weight.
- Control your alcohol intake.
- Don't smoke.
- Exercise as directed by your doctor.
- Lose weight if you are overweight or obese.[10,11]

Acute Coronary Syndrome

The major complication of cardiovascular disease is *acute coronary syndrome* (ACS). This term applies to several conditions and symptoms ranging from unstable angina to myocardial infarction (heart attack). ACS occurs when the heart does not get enough oxygenated blood flow. If the blood flow to the heart is cut off, a part of the heart will die, causing disability or death. Figure 3.5 shows damage to heart muscle from inadequate blood supply. ACS is the cause of sudden cardiac arrest in most adult victims.

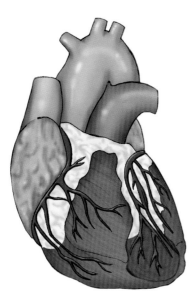

Figure 3.5   Damage to heart muscle.

Signs and Symptoms

There is a wide range, from slight to severe:

- Chest pain or a dull discomfort behind the breastbone that may or may not spread to the arms, back, neck, jaw, or stomach
- Shortness of breath
- Weakness, nausea, dizziness
- Heavy sweating
- Fear of impending doom (feeling like something extremely bad is going to happen but not sure what)
- Uncertainty and embarrassment
- Denial (victim often refuses to accept or believe he or she may be having a heart attack, which can delay treatment and increase the risk of death)

Treatment Guidelines

1. Have the victim sit down and rest quietly.
2. Loosen any tight clothing.
3. If the victim has a known heart condition, help the person take his or her medication. Usually this is nitroglycerin, placed or sprayed under the tongue.
4. If chest discomfort or pain does not improve or worsens 5 minutes after one dose has been taken, call 9-1-1 immediately.[12]
5. If the victim does not have a history of aspirin allergy, the 9-1-1 operator may recommend that the victim chew an aspirin while awaiting the arrival of EMS providers.

CAUTION!

The absence of chest pain, especially in people with diabetes, women, and the elderly, does not mean that the victim is not at risk. Unusual symptoms of a heart attack include headache, ringing in the ears, dizziness, hiccups, and belching. **Do not** downplay the seriousness of the potential problem.

6. If an aspirin is recommended, help the victim take it. The usual dose is a half or whole adult aspirin tablet (162 to 325 milligrams) chewed and swallowed.

7. If it's available and you are properly trained, give emergency oxygen.

8. Comfort, calm, and reassure the victim until EMS arrives.

9. If the victim becomes unresponsive and is not breathing normally, start CPR.

Stroke

A *stroke* happens when the blood supply to part of the brain is suddenly interrupted or when a blood vessel in the brain bursts, spilling blood into the spaces surrounding brain cells. Brain cells die when they no longer receive oxygen and nutrients from the blood or there is sudden bleeding into or around the brain (see figure 3.6).[13] Limiting the extent of brain damage caused by a stroke depends on rapid diagnosis and treatment in the hospital. This requires the victim, family members, or bystanders to quickly recognize the signs and symptoms of stroke and activate EMS.[14] To reduce brain injury and ensure the best recovery, EMS must be rapidly dispatched, you must quickly identify the potential stroke victim, and you must rapidly notify and transport the victim to a designated stroke center, if available.

Risk factors for stroke include the following:

- High blood pressure
- Diabetes
- Smoking
- High cholesterol level
- Heart disease

Signs and Symptoms[15]

- *Sudden* numbness or weakness of the face, an arm, or a leg, especially on one side of the body
- *Sudden* confusion, trouble speaking, or trouble understanding
- *Sudden* trouble seeing in one or both eyes
- *Sudden* trouble walking, dizziness, loss of balance, or loss of coordination
- *Sudden*, severe headache
- Ministroke (transient ischemic attack, or TIA): same symptoms as a stroke, but it lasts for only a few minutes

Note: Victims of stroke are sometimes mistaken for being drunk.

Treatment Guidelines

If you suspect a stroke, ask the victim to do the following:

1. Smile
2. Raise both arms
3. Speak a simple sentence

If the victim has any trouble with these tasks, he or she may be having a stroke. Alert EMS or initiate your emergency action plan immediately. If it's available and you are properly trained, give emergency oxygen. Comfort, calm, and reassure the victim.

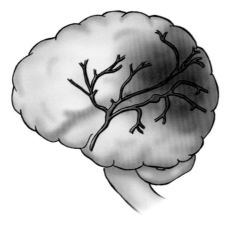

Figure 3.6 Damage to brain from stroke.

CAUTION!

Stroke treatments are time sensitive!

Sudden Cardiac Arrest

Sudden cardiac arrest (SCA) is one of the leading causes of death among adults in North America.[16] SCA occurs when the heart's electrical system malfunctions and the heart abruptly stops working without warning. When SCA occurs, most victims have an abnormal heart rhythm known as *ventricular fibrillation* (VF). The most common cause of VF is a poor supply of oxygen to the heart, most commonly caused by a heart attack.[17] After a heart attack, low oxygen can cause the heart's natural electronic signals to become disorganized. This causes twitching of the heart muscle (VF) and prevents coordinated contraction. The heart stops pumping blood and oxygen to itself and to the brain. The lack of blood flow and oxygen supply to the brain causes the victim to lose consciousness immediately. Unless a shock is delivered to the heart to restore its regular rhythm, brain death can occur within minutes.

SCA often occurs in active, outwardly healthy people with no known heart disease or other health problems. A victim of SCA may look like the man in figure 3.7. However, most victims have heart diseases or other health problems. The most important risk factors are a previous heart attack and coronary artery disease (CAD, narrowed or blocked arteries supplying blood to the heart).[18]

An automated external defibrillator (AED) is a small, portable computerized device that diagnoses and treats VF (see figure 3.8). It is attached with wires and pads to the chest of the victim. It checks the person's heart rhythm, decides if the rhythm is VF, and gives the heart an electric shock. If this shock is delivered promptly after collapse, many victims can survive without brain damage. If an AED is available, immediately attach it to the victim. Listen to and follow the machine's instructions.

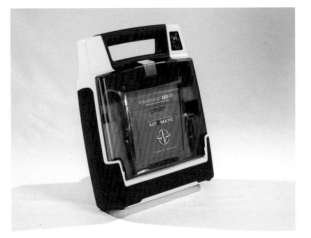

Figure 3.8   PowerHeart AED.
Courtesy Cardiac Science Corporation

Signs and Symptoms

- Sudden collapse without warning (some people may have a racing heartbeat or feel dizzy or faint)
- Unconsciousness or unresponsiveness
- Abnormal grunting, gasping, or snoring noises
- Looks dead

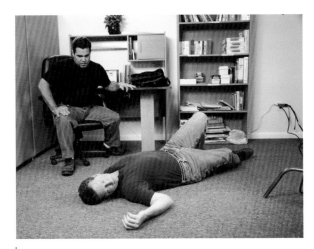

Figure 3.7   Cardiac arrest victim.

Sudden cardiac arrest should be treated with CPR and defibrillation with an AED as soon as possible.

Chain of Survival in Adults

The *chain of survival* is a concept used to communicate the key factors that must be in place if a victim is to survive sudden cardiac arrest (SCA) from ventricular fibrillation.[19] The links in the chain of survival include early identification of SCA, early CPR, early defibrillation, and early advanced life support (ALS). See figure 3.9.

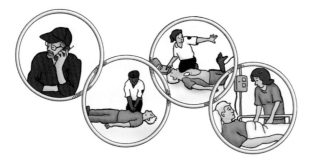

Figure 3.9   Chain of survival (adults).

- **Early identification.** Early identification of SCA and rapid activation of an emergency action plan or EMS involve assistance by emergency medical dispatch personnel who are specially trained to provide CPR instructions over the telephone. Dispatcher-assisted telephone CPR instruction can increase the proportion of SCA victims who receive CPR from bystanders. It also has been associated with improved survival.[20,21]

- **Early CPR.** Victims in cardiac arrest need immediate CPR. CPR provides a small but vital amount of blood flow to the heart and brain. CPR increases the chances that a shock from an AED will allow the heart to start working effectively.

- **Early defibrillation.** Survival rates are highest when immediate CPR is provided and defibrillation occurs within 3 to 5 minutes. When laypersons are equipped with and use AEDs, the highest survival rates are found in recreational complexes, public transportation facilities, and fitness centers.[22]

- **Early ALS.** Advanced life support involves medical procedures and medications used by paramedics, nurses, and doctors to manage a victim's vital signs and organ systems to increase the chances of survival and recovery.

If any one of these links is weak or missing, the result will be a poor chance of survival. Some organizations have added further links to the chain. These include making healthy choices that reduce the risk of heart attack, stroke, and injury and restoring the victim to the highest possible level of functional ability (early rehabilitation).[23]

Chain of Survival in Children

The chain of survival in children emphasizes prevention, basic CPR, early identification of an emergency with rapid activation of an emergency action plan (including EMS), and early pediatric advanced life support (see figure 3.10). Except for those with heart problems, a child's heart does not usually stop suddenly, as is often the case in adults. Rather, the heart slows and then stops only after the child has not been breathing for an extended time. Breathing stops because of a lack of oxygen in the blood. This can be caused by conditions such as injuries, drowning, and sudden infant death syndrome (SIDS).

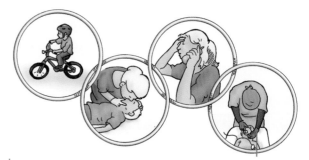

Figure 3.10   Chain of survival (children).

When an infant or child stops breathing but his or her heart continues to beat and rescue breathing is quickly provided, survival with normal (or near-normal) brain function is much higher, reportedly as much as 70%.[28] Giving infants and children rescue breaths that make the chest visibly rise is very important. When a rescuer finds a child unresponsive and not moving, he or she should give 2 minutes of CPR before calling 9-1-1 or attaching an AED. If another rescuer is present, he or she should activate the EMS or emergency action plan.

Prevention

- **Injuries.** Injury is a leading killer of children 14 and under worldwide. Most accidental injuries can be prevented by the use of simple safety measures.[24]
- **Drowning.** Death rates are highest in children less than 5 years of age. Pool fencing significantly reduces the risk of drowning. Pool fences with a secure, self-latching gate should be installed around all public, semipublic, and private pools.[25]
- **SIDS.** Placing infants on their backs to sleep and giving them a pacifier significantly reduces the risk of sudden infant death syndrome (SIDS).[26,27]

Emergency Action Steps

The emergency action steps are **assess, alert, and attend to the ABCDs.** They are intended to help you, as a CPR provider, respond to an emergency and manage life-threatening problems of the airway, breathing, and circulation of a victim of any age. CPR procedures differ for adults, children, and infants. Although no single factor can distinguish an infant from a child and a child from an adult, in order to simplify training, CPR guidelines use the age ranges shown in the following list:

Age Ranges for Adults, Children, and Infants

Adult = About 8 years of age and older

Child = About 1 to 8 years of age

Infant = Less than about 1 year of age

Note the use of the word *about* in the previous list. When it comes to basic life support, determining age can be difficult. Exactness is not necessary.

The following text contains detailed BLS and CPR recommendations for adults, children, and infants. For quick reference, refer to the Skill Guides on pages 82 to 86.

Assess

Assess the scene, then assess the victim.

- **Assess the scene.** Assess for safety. If the scene is not safe (see figure 3.11) or at any time becomes unsafe, **get out!**

- **Assess the victim.** If the scene is safe, pause for a moment as you approach the victim. What is your first impression? Is the victim lying

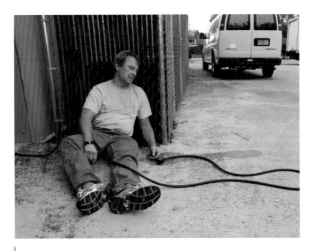

Figure 3.11   Unsafe scene.

still or moving around? Does skin color appear normal for the victim's ethnic group? Does it look difficult for the victim to breathe? Normal breathing is quiet and easy. Signs that basic life support or CPR may be needed include the following:

- Victim is not moving, is unresponsive, or looks dead.

- Skin tissue is bluish or ashen, especially around the lips.

- Skin tissue is cold and pale.

- Breathing is shallow, gasping, or absent.

- Pink or frothy discharge from mouth is present.

Gently tap or squeeze the victim's shoulder and ask, "Are you all right?" For an infant, you may tap the foot. Use the victim's name if you know it.

Alert

If the victim responds but is badly hurt, looks or acts very ill, or quickly gets worse, alert EMS (if you are in the United States or Canada call 9-1-1) or activate your emergency action plan. See figure 3.12. Use the following guidelines when you are responding in these situations.

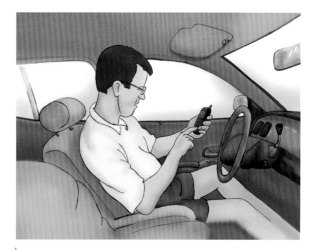

Figure 3.12   Alert EMS.

Adults (About 8 Years of Age and Older)

If you are alone and the victim is not moving or responding to your voice or touch, alert EMS (call 9-1-1) or activate your emergency action plan. Get an AED and emergency oxygen (if available) and return to the victim. When someone else is present, have him or her alert EMS while you begin CPR.

Children and Infants (Less Than About 8 Years of Age)

If a child or infant is unresponsive and is not moving, shout for help and immediately start CPR. Provide about 2 minutes of CPR before leaving the child to alert EMS (call 9-1-1) and get an AED and emergency oxygen (if available).

If the victim is an infant, it may be possible to carry the infant to a telephone as necessary while beginning the steps of CPR. When alerting EMS, be prepared to explain the exact situation. Many dispatchers today are trained to provide real-time instruction in CPR while simultaneously dispatching EMS to your location.

Attend to the ABCDs

The ABCDs are the action steps you should take when attending to the victim: airway, breathing, compression, and defibrillation. To properly attend to the victim, you must place him or her faceup on a firm, flat surface. If the victim is lying facedown, roll him or her over. Try to minimize turning or twisting of the head and neck.

A = Airway

The airway is the passageway between the mouth and lungs. It must be open so air can enter and leave the lungs freely. Blockage of the airway in an adult or child is commonly caused by the tongue. To open the airway, tilt the victim's head and lift the chin (see figure 3.13).

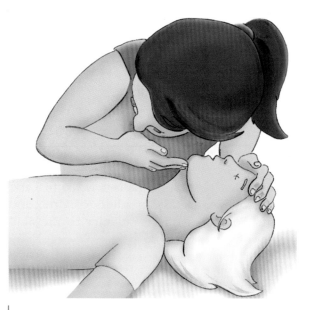

Figure 3.13   Tilt head, lift chin to open airway.

CAUTION!

Don't use your thumb to open the airway or press too hard on the soft area under the chin. Doing so can block the airway. Also, don't push the mouth completely closed.

B = Breathing

While keeping the airway open, look, listen, and feel for breathing for at least 5 seconds, but no more than 10 seconds.[29] Opening the airway might allow the victim to start breathing normally. If the victim is breathing normally, or starts breathing normally at any time, consider placing him or her in the recovery position. In this position, there is less chance of obstruction by the tongue and secretions. Make sure the victim's body position is stable so he or she does not roll onto the face or back. Also make sure there is no pressure on the chest that could make it more difficult to breathe. To prevent blood flow in the lower arm from being impaired, turn the victim to the opposite side if he or she is in the recovery position for more than 30 minutes.[30] If the victim is injured, use a modified recovery position called the HAINES method (described in chapter 2).

It may be difficult to determine whether the victim is breathing normally. *Normal* means effortless, quiet, and in a regular pattern. **Occasional gasps are not normal and are not capable of supplying the victim with enough oxygen to sustain life.** If the chest does not rise and fall and no air is exhaled, or if the victim is making strange gasping, noisy, snorting, or gurgling sounds and you are not positive that the victim is breathing normally, give two rescue breaths immediately. Give each breath in 1 second, and give enough air to make the chest visibly rise. If the victim's chest does not rise with the first rescue breath, reposition the head, make a better seal, and try again. **With children, you may have to try a couple of times to give two rescue breaths that make the chest visibly rise. It is critical that rescue breaths make the infant's or child's chest rise during CPR.**

Do not take deep breaths when performing rescue breathing. Taking deep breaths is unnecessary and may cause hyperventilation. If you suddenly feel breathless, have tiny prickling sensations, become dizzy, or have muscle spasms in your hands or feet, you are breathing too fast and deep. Slow down or have another person take over for you.

Air is often blown into the stomach instead of the lungs during rescue breathing. This can cause the victim to vomit and can limit lung movement, reducing the effectiveness of rescue breathing. To reduce the risk of inflating the victim's stomach, give each breath over one second, and give enough air to make the chest visibly rise, but no more than that. Allow the victim to exhale completely between breaths. If the victim vomits, turn the person on his or her side so he or she doesn't inhale the fluid.

When you perform rescue breathing, you should have a barrier such as a mask or face shield between you and the victim for protection against bloodborne pathogens. However, if necessary, you can provide mouth-to-mouth or mouth-to-nose breathing. You may at some time have to administer rescue breathing to someone who has a stoma (an opening at the front of the neck into the windpipe), and, when it is available, you may also need to administer emergency oxygen.

Mouth-to-Barrier Device Breathing

Masks and face shields allow you to perform rescue breathing without compromising your own health. These devices are usually available for all ages and sizes. They come with a replaceable one-way valve or filters to block contaminated fluids. All first aid kits should have at least one rescue breathing mask or face shield. Simple infection-control measures, including use of barrier devices, can reduce the risk of getting an infectious disease during CPR and CPR training.[31] Although the risk of getting a disease while giving BLS is extremely low, observing universal precautions for victims of all ages will make it lower. If you are a designated first aid or CPR provider at work, always observe universal precautions.

When using a mask, tilt the victim's head and lift the chin. Place the mask over the victim's mouth and nose. Place your mouth around the one-way valve on the mask and give two rescue breaths that make the chest visibly rise, but no more than that (see figure 3.14). Remove your

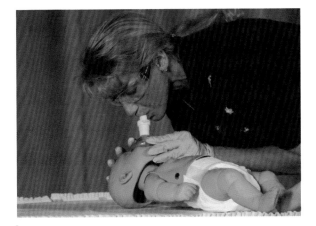

Figure 3.14 Rescue breathing with a mask.

mouth from the mask after each rescue breath and allow the victim to exhale.

When using a face shield, tilt the victim's head and lift the chin. Place the face shield over the victim's mouth and nose. Place your mouth on the face shield over the victim's mouth (see figure 3.15). Pinch the victim's nose either under or over the shield. Give two rescue breaths that make the chest visibly rise, but no more than that.

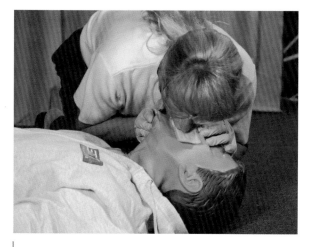

Figure 3.15   Rescue breathing with a face shield.

Mouth-to-Mouth Rescue Breathing

A rescuer's exhaled air contains about 17% oxygen and 4% carbon dioxide.[32] This oxygen concentration is sufficient to support life. To provide mouth-to-mouth rescue breathing for an adult, child, or large infant (see the next section for instructions on performing mouth-to-nose rescue breathing on small infants), hold the victim's airway open, pinch the nose, and make a seal with your mouth over the victim's mouth. Give two breaths that make the chest visibly rise, but no more than that. Because of the risk of poisoning, do not perform mouth-to-mouth rescue breathing for victims who have been poisoned by phosphorus compounds, including insecticides and herbicides.[33]

Mouth-to-Nose Rescue Breathing

When you have difficulty with mouth-to-mouth rescue breathing, you may want to use mouth-to-nose rescue breathing. Tilt the victim's head back with one hand and use the other hand to close the victim's mouth. Seal your lips around the victim's nose and give slow breaths that make the chest rise, but no more than that. If the victim is an infant, place your mouth over the infant's mouth and nose.

Stoma

A stoma is a surgical opening at the front of the neck that extends into the windpipe. When an adult or child with a stoma requires rescue breathing, give mouth-to-stoma rescue breaths (see figure 3.16). As an option, you can cover the stoma with a child-sized face mask, place your mouth around the one-way valve on the mask, and give rescue breaths.

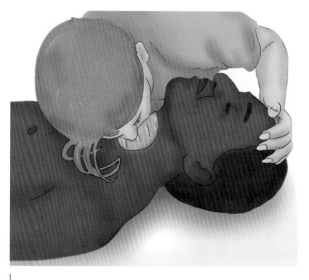

Figure 3.16   Rescue breathing through a stoma.

CAUTION!

Rescue breaths are important for victims in cardiac arrest, but rescuers should not give too many breaths or breaths that are too large or too forceful. Excessive breaths are unnecessary and harmful because they increase pressure in the victim's chest. This pressure decreases blood flow to and from the heart and reduces the already-marginal flow of blood and oxygen during CPR, thereby decreasing survival. **It is critical to avoid excessive rescue breaths.**

Emergency Oxygen

Emergency oxygen may be used during resuscitation without a prescription by anyone who has been properly trained.[34] A supply of emergency oxygen can be connected to a rescue breathing mask by tubing (see figure 3.17). This will significantly increase the amount of oxygen you can blow into the victim.

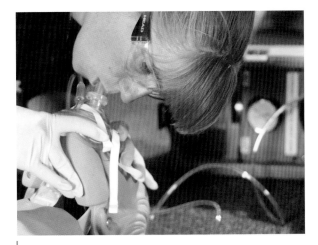

Figure 3.17 Mouth-to-mask breathing with emergency oxygen.

Even the best chest compression provides only about 25 to 33% of the normal blood and oxygen flow from the heart. This combination of low blood flow and low oxygen causes organs to fail and leads to death. Giving rescue breathing with emergency oxygen permits you to give a higher concentration of oxygen. Oxygen-rich breaths deliver critically needed oxygen to the heart and brain. For this reason, when emergency oxygen is available and you are trained to administer it, give it to both adults and children while providing mouth-to-mask rescue breathing. Administration of emergency oxygen is described in chapter 5 of this text. Learning to administer emergency oxygen may be part of the course in which you are enrolled.

C = Compressions

Compressions help keep a victim's blood circulating. In the past rescuers were told to check a victim's pulse before beginning compressions, but we now know that this is not a reliable way to check for circulation, and it is no longer recommended. Do not first check for a pulse or other signs of circulation. Instead, if an unresponsive victim is not breathing normally after you deliver two rescue breaths, immediately begin external chest compressions.

External Chest Compressions

External chest compression is a rhythmic application of pressure over the upper half of the breastbone. Chest compressions create blood flow through the heart and brain by increasing pressure inside the chest and arteries and by direct compression of the heart.[35] Creating and maintaining this pressure not only keep vital organs alive but also increase the chances that defibrillation will be successful.

Once chest compressions are started, it takes time to build up enough pressure to make blood flow. When chest compressions are stopped, the pressure and blood flow drop quickly. Thus, frequent interruption of chest compressions may contribute to poor survival rates.[36] For that reason, minimize interruptions in chest compressions during CPR.[37] Do not interrupt chest compressions to check for a pulse.

When another trained rescuer is available, it makes sense to take turns performing chest compressions and rescue breaths. Change positions at least every couple of minutes. Changing positions will help to prevent fatigue and maintain the quality of the chest compressions. Change positions quickly, in less than 5 seconds, so there is as little interruption in compression as possible. Continue CPR until a person with equal or more training takes over, EMS or an AED arrives, the victim shows signs of life, you are exhausted, or the scene becomes too dangerous to continue.

If you are unwilling or unable to provide rescue breathing, chest compressions alone are better than nothing. The best method of CPR is chest compressions combined with rescue breathing, and this is the recommended method.

Compression techniques are different for infants than they are for adults and children. Here are the techniques for each:

- **Adults and children.** To make blood flow to the heart and brain effective, you must place the victim faceup and lying flat on a firm surface. Place the heel of one hand in the center of the chest between the nipples. See figure 3.18.

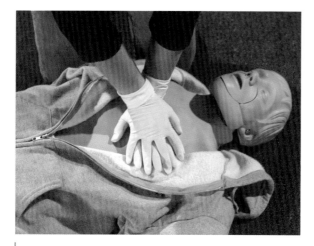

Figure 3.18   Adult: Push hard and fast.

Position your body so your shoulders are directly over your hands. Straighten your arms and lock your elbows. Put the other hand on top of the first. Your fingers can be straight or fastened together, but you should keep them off the chest. If you have difficulty pushing hard enough with this hand position, hold the wrist of the hand on the chest with the other hand and push down with both.

Use your upper-body weight to help compress the chest. **For a normal-sized adult,** push straight down on the chest approximately 1.5 to 2 inches (4 to 5 centimeters). **For a child,** use either one or two hands to compress the child's chest about one-third to one-half the depth of the chest (see figure 3.19). At the top of each compression, release pressure and completely remove your weight.

Chest compressions and relaxation should be about equal. Give 30 chest compressions at a speed of about 100 per minute. Keeping up the force, length, and speed of compressions helps create the best blood flow possible. **Do not** push over the lowest portion of the breastbone.

After 30 compressions, open the victim's airway and give two rescue breaths that make the chest visibly rise, but no more than that. Then return quickly to the chest and give 30 more compressions.

When adult chest compressions are given properly, you might hear an unpleasant sound like knuckles cracking. You might feel the breastbone fall in a bit. This is caused by cartilage or ribs cracking. Any damage done is not serious, so don't worry about it. Forceful external chest compression is critical if the victim is to survive without brain damage. In infants and toddlers, CPR rarely causes cracked ribs.[38]

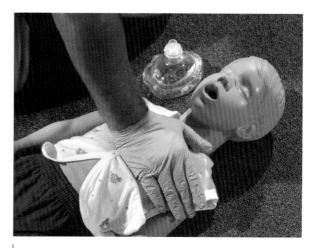

Figure 3.19   Child: Push hard and fast.

• **Infants.** Push the chest with two fingertips placed just below the nipple line (see figure 3.20). You may place your other hand under the infant's back to create a compression surface. Press down on the breastbone about one-third to one-half the depth of the infant's chest. After each compression, completely release the pressure on the breastbone and allow it to return to its normal position. Give 30 chest compressions at a speed of about 100 per minute.

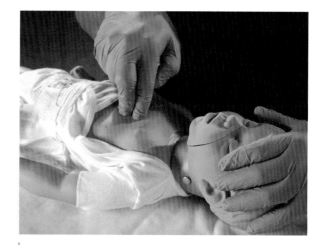

Figure 3.20   Infant: Push hard and fast.

D = Defibrillation

When sudden cardiac arrest occurs, most victims have an abnormal heart rhythm called *ventricular fibrillation* (VF). If the heart can be shocked quickly with an AED, a normal heart rhythm may be restored. No more than 3 minutes from collapse to defibrillation is necessary for achieving the highest survival rates.[39] The following are some precautions that you must take before attaching the AED and the procedures for using the AED for adults and children. Defibrillation is not recommended for infants. Also presented are the steps to using an AED, troubleshooting and maintenance of the AED, and how the AED fits into an overall program of high-quality care.

Preparations Before AED Use

Before attaching the AED, quickly check for the following situations:

- **Chest hair.** If the victim's chest is covered with hair, it may prevent the electrode pads from making effective contact with the skin. If the AED voice prompt continues to say, "Check pads" or something similar after you attach the pads, quickly remove the pads, tearing out the hair under them. Apply a second set of electrodes. If the problem continues, quickly shave the chest in the area of the pads and attach another set of electrodes.

- **Water.** Move the victim out of freestanding fresh- or saltwater before attaching the AED. Water or sweat on the victim's chest may also conduct energy from one electrode pad to the other, reducing the potential for a successful shock. If the victim's chest is wet, sweaty, or dirty, quickly clean and dry it before attaching the AED.

- **Medication patches.** Remove medication patches and wipe the skin area clean before attaching the AED electrode pads. Medication patches left in place may block the shock and can cause small burns to the skin.

- **Implanted medical devices.** Pacemakers and implantable cardioverter defibrillators (ICDs) can interfere with the use of an AED. Place electrode pads at least 1 inch (2.5 centimeters) away from an implanted device. Look for a lump beneath the skin of the upper chest or abdomen. If the victim is receiving internal shocks from the ICD (which looks similar to muscles contracting from external shocks from an AED), allow 30 to 60 seconds for the ICD to complete its cycle before attaching the AED. Rescuers touching the victim will not be harmed if the implanted device discharges.[42]

- **Oxygen.** Do not use oxygen when delivering shocks with an AED. There have been reports of victims and their bedding being set on fire during defibrillation.[43] The oxygen concentration necessary to produce ignition will typically extend less than a foot (30 centimeters) in any direction and will quickly disperse when removed. Therefore, you should remove the mask and place it several feet from the victim or shut off the oxygen flow when delivering shocks. Leaving a device that continues to discharge oxygen near the victim's head before defibrillation is dangerous.[44]

Metal surfaces pose no shock hazard to either you or the victim, and cell phones do not interfere with the AED. Always follow the manufacturer's recommended safety precautions.

AED Use for Adults

Expose the victim's chest, turn on the AED, and immediately attach it to the victim. Whenever possible, position it next to the rescuer who will be operating it. If feasible, continue CPR while the pads are being applied. Listen carefully and follow the machine's instructions. See figure 3.21.

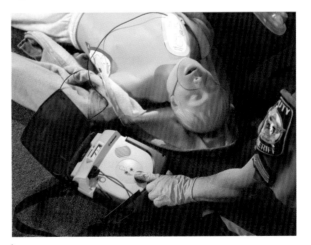

Figure 3.21 Defibrillation.

AED Use for Children

Although ventricular fibrillation is an uncommon cause of cardiac arrest in infants, it occurs more frequently with age. AEDs may be used on children older than 1 year who have no signs of life. Figure 3.22 shows a pediatric defibrillator. Some AED pads may require that the rescuer place one pad on the child's chest and one on the back. Always look at the pictures on the pads and place them as shown. The rescuer may need to use different cables or insert a key or turn a switch to deliver a lower amount of electricity for a child. If a child-specific AED is not available, use a standard AED.[40,41]

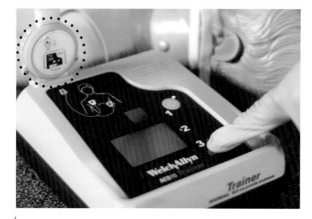

Figure 3.22   AED with Pediatric Energy Reducer.
Courtesy Welch Allyn®, Inc.

Attaching and Operating an AED

If there is an AED in your workplace or community, you should become very familiar with it so you and other rescuers can operate it during an emergency. Medical emergencies are emotionally distressing and often chaotic. Familiarity with the AED (and other emergency equipment) will help you remain calm and confident and act sensibly.

AEDs are very easy to use. Research has shown that people can use AEDs adequately and safely without **any** instruction.[45-47] This includes sixth-grade students using an AED for the first time in a simulated cardiac arrest. These untrained students were able to use the AED safely and only moderately slower than paramedics.[48] Training is still recommended. Getting as little as 15 minutes of AED training has been shown to significantly improve the ability to operate it.[49,50] Rescuers should practice together as a team to make sure their actions are well timed and effective. ASHI recommends skill review and practice drills every 6 months. An AED program should be part of an overall system of quality assurance that includes medical oversight, training, data collection, and evaluation.

Many different brands of AEDs exist, but the same basic steps apply to all of them. If the victim is unresponsive and not breathing normally, follow these steps:

1. Turn on the AED. Turning on the AED activates the voice prompts. Bare the victim's chest.

2. Follow the voice and visual prompts. Remove the disposable electrode pads from the packaging. Make sure to choose the correct pads (adult or child). **Do not use child pads or systems for an adult.** Look at the graphic images on each electrode as a guide for proper pad placement. Remove the self-adhesive backing and attach the electrodes to the victim's bare chest. Make sure the electrode attaches firmly to the skin. Do not apply the pad over a female's breast, because it might decrease effectiveness.[51] Most AEDs will automatically begin to analyze a victim's heart rhythm when the electrodes are fully attached and plugged into the device. Some will prompt you to push a button to analyze. Ensure that nobody touches the victim while the AED is analyzing the heart rhythm.

3. Follow procedures for shock or no shock. If a shock is indicated, check to make sure no one is touching the victim. Loudly say, "Clear!" or something similar. Push the shock button and immediately resume chest compressions. If no shock is indicated, immediately resume chest compressions. Perform 5 cycles of 30 compressions and 2 breaths. Continue as directed by the AED.

Research shows that errors by AED operators do occur. These include interference in AED operation by unnecessary movement (CPR), inappropriately turning the AED off, pads falling off or being disconnected, shockable rhythm not shocked, inappropriate shock delivered, and interference from movement other than CPR.[52,53] Very few cardiac rhythms are mismanaged by AEDs. AED operators must listen carefully and follow the AED's prompts.

Troubleshooting an AED

If an AED detects a problem during use, a voice or visual prompt, screen message, or lit icon will be displayed. Stay calm and do what the AED tells you to do. Here are some examples:

- If a message indicating motion occurs, make sure the cables are not being moved around.

- If a message regarding the battery is displayed, the battery power is probably low. The AED will prompt you to change the battery.

Maintenance and Quality Assurance

AEDs perform regular self-tests to make sure they are ready for use. If an AED fails a self-test,

it will alert you with an audible prompt. Contact authorized service personnel immediately. Inspect AEDs monthly. If the AED has a visual status indicator, check it to make sure it shows the device is operational. Examine the expiration dates on pad packages and spare batteries and inspect the AED for obvious damage. Make sure the battery and a replacement battery (or batteries) are fully operational and ready to use.

Store AEDs with the necessary equipment to respond to a cardiac arrest. The equipment should include the following, at a minimum:

- Personal protective equipment (rescue breathing shield or mask and disposable gloves)

- Utility scissors (to cut clothing and expose chest)

- A disposable razor (to shave a hairy chest)

- Disposable towels (to dry the chest)

- A plastic biohazard bag (to dispose of used supplies)

CPR and AED for Adults

Emergency Action Steps

1. **Assess scene.** If the scene is not safe or at any time becomes unsafe, **get out!**
2. **Assess victim.** Not moving? No response?
3. **Alert.** Shout for help. No help? Alert EMS or activate your emergency action plan. Get the AED and oxygen.
4. **Attend to the ABCDs.**

A = Airway

Open the airway. Tilt head and lift chin.

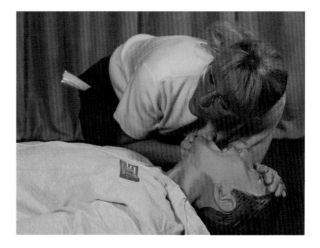

B = Breathing

- Look, listen, and feel for 5, but no more than 10, seconds.
- If the victim is not breathing normally, place a barrier or mask over the victim's mouth or nose.
- Give 2 breaths (each over 1 second long). Make the victim's chest visibly rise, but no more than that.

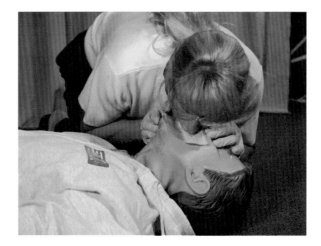

C = Compressions

- Give 30 chest compressions, 2 rescue breaths (30:2). Repeat.
  - Push on the middle of the chest between the nipples.
  - Push hard and fast (100 times per minute) 1.5 to 2 inches deep (4 to 5 centimeters).
  - Allow the chest to recoil completely. Minimize interruptions.
  - Continue 30:2 until an AED or EMS or advanced providers arrive or the victim shows signs of life.

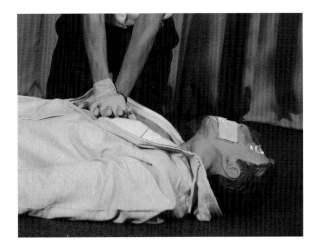

D = Defibrillation

- Expose the chest and turn on the AED. Select and attach the **adult** pads. Follow the AED voice prompts.
  - **Shock** advised: **Clear** and give 1 shock. Immediately resume chest compressions.
  - **No shock** advised: Immediately resume chest compressions.
- Continue 30 compressions, 2 breaths × 5 cycles. Check rhythm. Continue as directed by the AED.

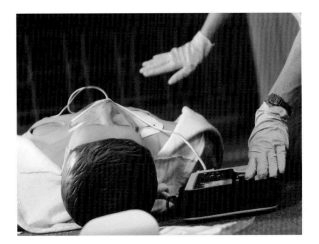

CPR and AED for Children

Emergency Action Steps

1. **Assess scene.** If the scene is not safe or at any time becomes unsafe, **get out!**
2. **Assess victim.** Not moving? No response?
3. **Alert.** Shout for help. Send help to alert EMS, activate the emergency action plan, and get the AED and oxygen.
4. **Attend to the ABCDs.**

A = Airway

Open the airway. Tilt head and lift chin.

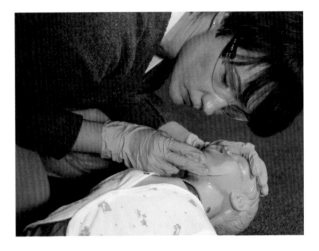

B = Breathing

- Look, listen, and feel for 5, but no more than 10, seconds.
- If the victim is not breathing, place a barrier or mask over the victim's mouth or nose.
- Give 2 breaths (each over 1 second long). Make the victim's chest visibly rise, but no more than that.

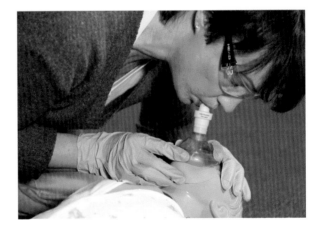

C = Compressions

- Give 30 chest compressions, 2 rescue breaths. Repeat.
  - Push on the middle of the chest between the nipples.
  - Push hard and fast (100 times per min), one-third to one-half the depth of the chest.
  - Allow the chest to recoil completely. Minimize interruptions.
  - Continue 30:2. If alone, alert EMS after 5 cycles.

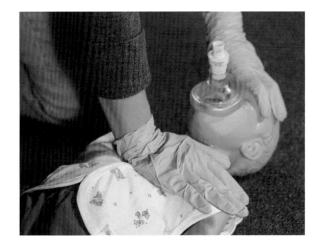

D = Defibrillation

- Expose the chest and turn on the AED. Select and attach the **child** pads or system (if not available, use the adult pads or system).
- Follow the voice prompts.
  - **Shock** advised: Clear and give 1 shock. Immediately resume chest compressions.
  - **No shock** advised: Immediately resume chest compressions.
- Continue 30 compressions, 2 breaths × 5 cycles. Check rhythm. Continue as directed by the AED.

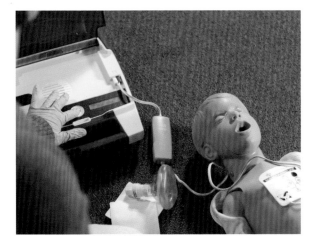

CPR for Infants

Emergency Action Steps

1. **Assess scene.** If the scene is not safe or at any time becomes unsafe, **get out!**
2. **Assess victim.** Not moving? No response?
3. **Alert.** Shout for help. Send help to alert EMS, activate the emergency action plan, and get the oxygen.
4. **Attend to the ABCs.**

A = Airway

Open the airway. Tilt head and lift chin.

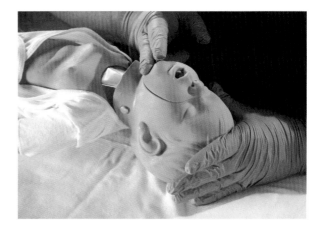

B = Breathing

- Look, listen, and feel for 5, but no more than 10, seconds.
- If there is no breathing, place a barrier or mask over the victim's mouth and nose.
- Give 2 breaths (each over 1 second long). Make the victim's chest visibly rise, but no more than that.

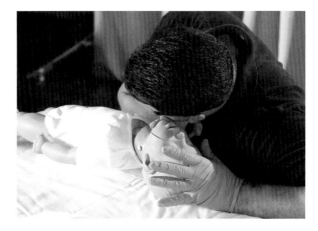

C = Compressions

- Give 30 chest compressions, 2 rescue breaths. Repeat.
  - Use 2 fingertips, just below the nipples.
  - Push hard and fast (100 times per minute), one-third to one-half the depth of the chest.
  - Allow the chest to recoil completely. Minimize interruptions.
  - Continue 30:2. If alone, alert EMS after 5 cycles.

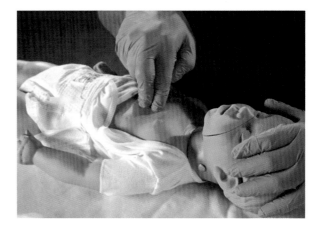

Summary of Basic Life Support Procedures

Table 3.1 summarizes the BLS procedures for adults, children, and infants.

Table 3.1 Basic Life Support Procedures

	Adult (over 8 years)	Child (1 to 8 years)	Infant (under 1 year)
Assess			
Scene	If the scene is not safe or at any time becomes unsafe, **get out!**	If the scene is not safe or at any time becomes unsafe, **get out!**	If the scene is not safe or at any time becomes unsafe, **get out!**
Victim	Check for response. If victim is unresponsive or not moving . . .	Check for response. If victim is unresponsive or not moving . . .	Check for response. If victim is unresponsive or not moving . . .
Alert: EMS or emergency action plan.	**Alert** as soon as victim is found.	Give about 5 cycles of CPR, then **alert.**	Give about 5 cycles of CPR, then **alert.**
Attend to the ABCDs.			
Airway: Open airway.	Tilt head, lift chin.	Tilt head, lift chin.	Tilt head, lift chin.
Breathing: Look, listen, and feel for at least 5, but no more than 10, seconds.	**Initial:** Give 2 rescue breaths. Give each breath in 1 second. Make chest visibly rise.	**Initial:** Give 2 rescue breaths. Give each breath in 1 second. Make chest visibly rise.	**Initial:** Give 2 rescue breaths. Give each breath in 1 second. Make chest visibly rise.
Compressions			
Position	In center of chest, between nipples, use 2 hands.	In center of chest, between nipples, use 1 or 2 hands.	Use 2 fingertips, just below nipple line.
Method	Hard, fast, complete recoil, minimize interruption.	Hard, fast, complete recoil, minimize interruption.	Hard, fast, complete recoil, minimize interruption.
Depth	1.5 to 2 inches (4 to 5 centimeters).	About one-third to one-half depth of chest.	About one-third to one-half depth of chest.
Speed	About 100 times a minute.	About 100 times a minute.	About 100 times a minute.
Ratio	30:2	30:2	30:2
Defibrillation (AED)			
Operation	Expose chest, turn on AED. Select and attach **adult** pads. Follow voice prompts.	Expose chest, turn on AED. Select and attach **child** pads or system. Follow voice prompts.	No recommendations.
Type	Standard AED. Do **not** use child system.	Use **child** pads or system. If not available, use a standard AED.	No recommendations.

Choking (Foreign-Body Airway Obstruction)

Coughing is the body's way of trying to remove a foreign object (such as food) from the throat. If coughing does not clear the object, then choking occurs. Choking is an emergency that will result in unconsciousness and brain death within minutes if left untreated.

Children are particularly at risk for choking because of the small size of their air passages, inexperience with chewing, and a natural tendency to put objects in their mouths. In children ages 5 to 14 years, the majority of choking episodes are associated with food, especially candy. See figure 3.23. For children ages 1 to 4 years, coins are involved in 18% of all choking-related emergencies.[54] Peanuts and other nuts also are common causes of choking.[55] Children under 3 years of age should never be fed nuts or other hard, crunchy foods.[56]

Adults commonly choke on large pieces of food, often while drinking alcohol. Elderly persons frequently choke on semisolid foods.[57] When the air

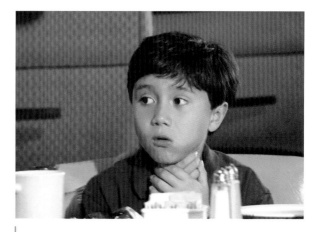

Figure 3.23   Child choking.

passages are blocked, the victim cannot breathe. Rapid first aid for choking can save a life. Table 3.2 shows the signs and symptoms and treatment guidelines for choking adults, children, and infants. Also see Skill Guides 4 and 5 on pages 90-91.

Table 3.2   Signs and Symptoms and Treatment for Choking

Adults and children older than 1 year

Air exchange is good (mild blockage)	
Signs and symptoms	Treatment guidelines
• Conscious or responsive • Can breathe in and out and can speak • Strong coughing or gagging as food or liquid "goes down the wrong pipe" • May hear high-pitched, squeaking, or whistling noise (wheezing) between strong coughs	• Encourage the victim to cough. • Stay with the victim. • Watch closely. • Be ready to take action if the symptoms worsen. • If blockage continues, alert EMS. *Note:* An incomplete obstruction of the airway may have less severe symptoms and be confused with other causes of upper-airway obstruction, such as reactive airway disease (asthma) or croup. If the victim is coughing forcefully, help him or her into a comfortable position. Call EMS or activate your emergency action plan.

Air exchange is poor or nonexistent (severe blockage)		
	Signs and symptoms	Treatment guidelines
Responsive	• Clutches throat • Cannot cough or make any sound • Blue lips, nails, skin	• Quickly ask, "Are you choking?" If the victim nods yes or is unable to speak, cough, or cry, **act quickly!** • Stand behind an adult or kneel behind a child. • Make a fist. Place the thumb side of your fist against the victim's abdomen, just above the navel. • Give quick inward and upward thrusts until the object is expelled or the victim becomes unresponsive. (See Skill Guide 4.)

Late stages of pregnancy or obese		• Perform chest thrusts. Stand behind the victim. • Place your arms under the victim's armpits, encircling the chest. Place the thumb side of your fist on the middle of the sternum. • Grasp your fist with your other hand and thrust backward. Continue until the object is expelled or the victim becomes unresponsive.
Self		• Give yourself abdominal thrusts until the object is expelled. • If that does not work, press your abdomen quickly over any firm surface (back of a chair, side of a table).
Unresponsive		• Carefully get the victim to the ground and immediately alert EMS or activate emergency action plan. • Open the airway. Remove the object if you see it. Begin CPR. • Each time the airway is opened for rescue breaths, look for an object in the victim's throat. If you see it, remove it. • Continue CPR until the AED or EMS arrives or the victim shows signs of life.

Caution!

Abdominal thrusts have been associated with severe and fatal complications. Complications may occur even when abdominal thrusts are performed correctly. **Do not** perform the Heimlich maneuver on an adult or child unless it is necessary. A victim who had an airway obstruction that was removed by abdominal or chest thrusts should be evaluated by EMS and seen by a physician to ensure no internal injuries resulted from the event.

Infants

Air exchange is good (mild blockage)		
	Signs and symptoms	**Treatment guidelines**
Responsive	• Can breathe in and out • Crying, gagging • Strong coughing • May hear high-pitched whistling or squeaking noise (wheezing) between strong coughs	• Stay with the victim. • Watch closely. • Be ready to take action if the symptoms worsen. • If blockage continues, alert EMS.
Air exchange is poor or nonexistent (severe blockage)		
Responsive	• Cannot cough or make any sound • Blue lips, nails, skin • Passing out	• Keep the infant's head lower than the chest. • Give 5 back slaps between the shoulder blades with enough force to expel the object. • Turn the infant faceup onto your lap or thigh. • Give 5 downward chest thrusts just below the nipple line with enough force to expel the object. • Repeat until the object is expelled or the infant becomes unresponsive.
Unresponsive		• Place the infant on a firm, flat surface. • Open the airway. Remove the object if you see it. • Begin CPR. • Each time the airway is opened for rescue breaths, look for an object in the infant's throat. If you see it, remove it. • Continue CPR for about 2 minutes (5 cycles). Alert EMS or activate emergency action plan.

Caution!

The Heimlich maneuver is not recommended for infants because you may damage internal organs. An infant who had an airway obstruction that was removed by back slaps or chest thrusts should be evaluated by EMS and seen by a physician to ensure no internal injuries resulted from the event.

Adult or Child Choking: Severe Blockage

Emergency Action Steps

Assess, alert, and attend to the ABCs.

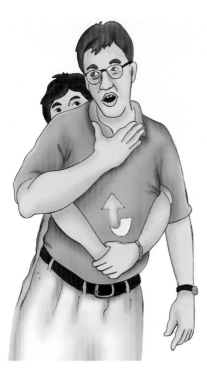

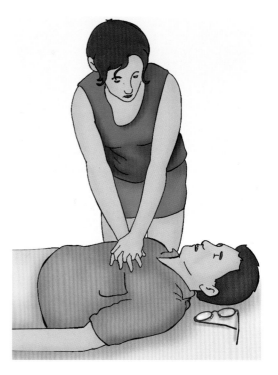

Responsive

- Victim is clutching throat and cannot cough or make any sound.
- Quickly ask, "Are you choking?"
- If the victim nods yes or is unable to speak, cough, or cry, act quickly.
- Stand behind an adult or kneel behind a child.
- Make a fist. Place the thumb side against the victim's abdomen, just above the navel.
- Give quick inward and upward thrusts until the object is expelled or the victim becomes unresponsive.

Unresponsive

- Carefully get the victim to the ground, immediately activate EMS, or activate your emergency action plan. If you are alone with a child, give about 5 cycles (2 minutes) of CPR, then alert EMS.
- Open the airway. Remove the object if you see it. Begin CPR.
- Each time you open the airway for rescue breaths, look for an object in the victim's throat. If you see it, remove it.
- Continue CPR until the AED or EMS arrives or the victim shows signs of life.

Infant Choking: Severe Blockage

Emergency Action Steps

Assess, alert, and attend to the ABCs.

Responsive

- Infant cannot cough, cry, or make any sound.
- Rest the infant facedown on your forearm. Place your forearm on your lap or thigh.
- Keep the infant's head lower than the chest. Support the head and jaw with your hand.
- Give 5 back slaps between the shoulder blades with enough force to expel the object.
- Support the head and neck and turn the infant over (faceup) onto your lap or thigh.
- Give 5 downward chest thrusts just below the nipple line with enough force to expel the object.
- Repeat until the object is expelled or the infant becomes unresponsive.

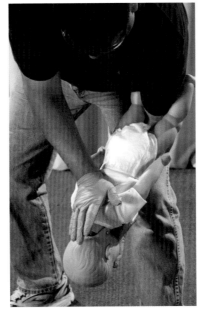
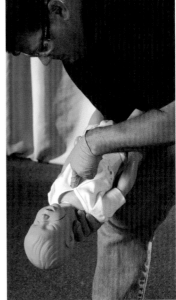

Unresponsive

- Place the infant on a firm, flat surface.
- Open the airway. Remove the object if you see it.
- Begin CPR.
- Each time you open the airway for rescue breaths, look for an object in the infant's throat. If you see it, remove it.
- Continue CPR for about 2 minutes (5 cycles). Alert EMS or activate your emergency action plan.

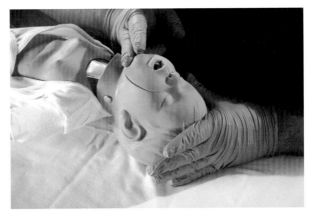

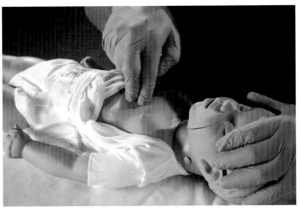

Psychological and Legal Aspects of Providing Basic Life Support

Evidence exists that persons trained in CPR are often unwilling to perform it—both in and outside of a hospital setting. They give a variety of reasons, including fear of hurting the victim, fear of performing the skills incorrectly, fear of liability, and fear of disease.[58,59] Remember that the risk of getting disease while giving CPR is extremely low, and observing universal precautions for victims of all ages will make it lower. The following are some of the psychological and legal aspects of providing basic life support.

Psychological Aspects

Fear is a common and intense emotion at the time of a medical emergency. Fortunately, much of the fear associated with CPR can be reduced through regular participation in training that focuses on simple, practical skills and confidence building. Still, when rescuers at all levels attempt resuscitation, they have a wide range of negative reactions and emotional stress.[60-63] Failed resuscitation attempts often leave those who infrequently perform resuscitation with feelings of guilt and failure when CPR was not done correctly.[64] This distress is normal and usually temporary.

Rib and breastbone fractures do occur frequently during chest compressions in adult CPR, but they are not major complications.[65] In infants and toddlers, CPR rarely causes such injuries.[66] Although CPR should be done correctly, it is helpful to remember that a person in cardiac arrest is dead (without breathing or a pulse). It is difficult to make the person "worse." The root of the word *resuscitate* is from the Latin *revivere,* which means "to live again." Rescuers who perform good CPR in a good-faith effort to give the victim a chance to live again should not hold themselves responsible when that attempt does not restore life fully—or at all. Mistakes in resuscitation may reduce the chances for successfully resuscitating victims, but the mistakes do not kill

Table 3.3   Traumatic Stress Reactions

	Signs and symptoms	Recommendations
During the incident	<ul><li>Anxiety or worry</li><li>Trembling or shaking</li><li>Sweating</li><li>Fast breathing</li><li>Pounding heartbeat, shock, anger</li><li>Excitement, intense fear</li><li>Nausea</li></ul>	<ul><li>Remain calm and act sensibly.</li><li>Accept your own limitations as a rescuer.</li></ul>
After the incident	<ul><li>Repeated thoughts or flashbacks of event</li><li>Worry about self or loved ones</li><li>Guilt for not having done more or better</li><li>Tense muscles, diarrhea or constipation, nausea or vomiting, headaches, fatigue</li><li>Avoiding reminders of incident</li><li>Easily startled</li><li>Lack of interest in usual activities</li><li>Sadness, feeling numb or detached</li><li>Sleep problems or nightmares</li><li>Problems concentrating</li><li>Hyperactive or depressed</li></ul>	<ul><li>Remind yourself that stress reactions are normal and will pass.</li><li>Get back into a normal routine as soon as possible.</li><li>Be kind to yourself. Allow yourself time to deal with memories of the incident.</li><li>Accept every person's right to his or her own feelings.</li><li>Keep what happened in a realistic perspective.</li><li>Exercise, eat, drink, and rest.</li><li>Have a connection to professional resources for continued care if necessary.</li></ul>

them. The majority of adult and child victims of cardiac arrest are not brought back to life.

Those who attempt CPR may also have traumatic stress reactions after they respond to a crisis. Traumatic stress reactions are a normal human response to a traumatic event and are usually temporary. Symptoms begin within minutes of the traumatic event and should disappear within hours or a couple days. Table 3.3 gives an

overview of the traumatic stress reactions that rescuers may have after a rescue event and recommendations for addressing those reactions.

Legal and Ethical Aspects

A few key legal and ethical principles are involved when you provide basic life support, which are described in table 3.4.

Table 3.4 Legal and Ethical Principles of BLS

Principle	Key points
Good Samaritan principle and laws	• Based on the Biblical story. Prevents a rescuer who has voluntarily helped a stranger in need from being sued for wrongdoing. • In most of North America you have no legal obligation to help a person in need.[a] Since governments want to encourage people to help others, they pass Good Samaritan laws (or apply the principle to common laws). • You are generally protected from liability as long as you are reasonably careful, act in good faith (not for reward), and do not provide care beyond your skill level. • If you decide to help an ill or injured person, you must not leave that person until someone with equal or more emergency training takes over (unless it becomes dangerous to stay).
Consent	• *Consent* means permission. A responsive adult must agree to receive first aid care. • *Expressed consent* means the victim gives his or her permission to receive care. To get consent, first identify yourself. Then tell the victim your level of training and ask if it's OK to help. • *Implied consent* means that permission to perform care on an unresponsive victim is assumed. This is based on the idea that a reasonable person would give permission to receive lifesaving care if he or she were able. • **Children:** Consent must be gained from a parent or legal guardian. When life-threatening situations exist and a parent or legal guardian is not available, care should be given based on implied consent. • **Elderly:** If suffering from a disturbance in normal mental functioning, such as Alzheimer's disease, a victim may not understand your request for consent. Consent must be gained from a family member or legal guardian.
Duty to act	• *Duty to act* means a legal obligation to do something. • Those with a duty to act are typically designated responders at work or state-licensed health care providers who are required to provide emergency medical care, including CPR, as part of their job. However, an off-duty response would generally be considered a Good Samaritan act (voluntary). • If you are not a designated responder at work or a state-licensed health care provider, generally you do not have a duty to act.

(continued)

Table 3.4 *(continued)*

Principle	Key points

Starting and stopping CPR	Start CPR for all victims of cardiac arrest unless
	
	• signs of irreversible death are present, including the following:
	  - Rigor mortis (limbs of the corpse are stiff and impossible to move)
	  - Lividity (settling of blood in the lower portions of the body, causing a purplish red discoloration)
	  - Conditions incompatible with life (decomposition, decapitation, massive head injury)
	• providing CPR would put the rescuer in danger of injury,
	• victim has a valid DNR order (see section at end of table), or
	• there are many victims (for example, in a catastrophic natural disaster or terrorist attack).
	
	A victim who is not breathing after two attempts to open the airway is considered dead. This is because the time required to provide rescue breathing and external chest compressions is not justified when there are many victims needing first aid.
	
	Do not stop CPR until any of the following conditions occur:
	• A person with equal or more training takes over.
	• EMS arrives or the victim shows signs of life.
	• You are exhausted.
	• The scene becomes too dangerous to continue.
	
	Note: Except when death is obvious, irreversible brain damage or brain death cannot be reliably assessed or predicted.[67] Rescuers should never make an impulsive decision about the present or future quality of life of a cardiac arrest victim because such decisions are often incorrect.

Advance directives and living wills	• These are documents authorized by state law and are usually witnessed or notarized. They are also called a *durable power of attorney*. • The documents allow a person to appoint someone as his or her representative to make decisions on resuscitation and continued life support if the person has lost his or her decision-making capacity (for example, if he or she is in a coma). • Advance directives are statements about what you want done or not done if you can't speak for yourself. Everyone should have an advance directive. An accident or serious illness can happen suddenly, and if you already have a signed advance directive, your wishes are more likely to be followed. • Laws about advance directives are different in each state. You should be aware of the laws in your state.
Do not resuscitate (DNR) or do not attempt resuscitation (DNAR) orders	• The DNR or DNAR order is a type of advance directive. This is a specific request not to have CPR if your heart stops or if you stop breathing. • In the United States, a doctor's order is required for withholding CPR. Therefore, unless you have a DNR order, EMS providers and hospital staff will attempt to resuscitate you under the principle of implied consent. • People who are not likely to benefit from CPR and may want a DNR order include victims with terminal conditions from which they are unlikely to recover. • As with the living will, it's best to consider your wishes for resuscitation early, before you are very sick and unable to make your own decisions.

[a] There are exceptions. Two U.S. states (Vermont and Minnesota) and one Canadian province (Quebec) have failure-to-act laws that require all citizens to assist a victim in need as long as they don't endanger their own lives.

Special Conditions

The following conditions may or may not require changes in standard CPR procedures. However, each condition requires some special consideration. See table 3.5 for those specific considerations.

Table 3.5 Specific Considerations for Special Conditions

Condition	Changes or special considerations
Pregnancy	**Assess scene and victim: no change. A = airway: no change. B = breathing: no change. C = compressions: change.** Chest compressions may not be effective when a woman who is 6 months pregnant or more is lying flat on her back. This is because the baby puts pressure on a major vein that returns blood to the heart. If possible, prop up the woman slightly on her left side using a rolled blanket (or something similar) when performing chest compressions. This reduces the pressure and provides the most blood flow to the mother and baby. Perform chest compressions higher on the breastbone, slightly above the center. **D = defibrillation: no change.**
Hypothermia	**Assess scene and victim: change.** Get inside or out of the wind. Prevent additional heat loss by removing wet clothes and insulating the victim from further exposure. If the body is frozen solid, nose and mouth are blocked with ice and chest compression is impossible, do not start CPR. **A = airway: no change. B = breathing: no change. C = compressions: no change. D = defibrillation: change.** If the patient does not respond to one shock, focus on continuing CPR and rewarming the victim to a range of 86 to 89.6 °F (30 to 32 °C) before repeating a defibrillation attempt.
Submersion or near drowning	**Assess scene and victim: change.** Caution! The scene may be unsafe (waves, currents, cold water, bad weather). Proper training and use of personal lifesaving equipment, such as rescue devices and personal flotation devices, are critical for a safe rescue. If a boat or other vessel is available, get the victim into it. If no boat is available, get the victim to the shore. Start BLS or CPR if indicated, as soon as it is safe to do so. **A = airway: no change. B = breathing: change.** Expect vomiting. When it occurs, turn the victim to the side and remove the vomit with a sweep of a gloved finger or cloth. If a head, neck, or back injury is suspected, use the HAINES method or roll the victim like a log. Minimize movement. Avoid twisting the head, neck, or back. Do not attempt to drain water from the lungs using abdominal thrusts or the Heimlich maneuver. It is unnecessary and potentially dangerous. **C= compressions: no change. D = defibrillation: change.** Move the victim out of freestanding water and dry the chest before attaching an AED.
Electric shock	**Assess scene and victim: change.** Consider any fallen or broken wire extremely dangerous. Do not touch (or allow your clothing to touch) a wire, victim, or vehicle that is possibly energized. Do not approach within 8 feet (2.4 meters) of it. Notify the local utility company and have trained personnel sent to the scene. Metal or cable guardrails, steel wire fences, and telephone lines may be energized by a fallen wire and may carry the current 1 mile (1.6 kilometers) or more from the point of contact. **Never** attempt to handle wires yourself unless you are properly trained and equipped.[68] Start BLS or CPR, if indicated, as soon as it is safe to do so. **A = airway: no change. B = breathing: no change. C = compressions: no change. D = defibrillation: no change.**
Lightning strike	**Assess scene and victim: change.** When multiple victims are struck by lightning at the same time, give the highest priority to those without signs of life. Start BLS or CPR, if indicated, as soon as it is safe to do so. Because many victims are young, they have a good chance for survival if CPR is given immediately. Remove smoldering clothing, shoes, and belts to prevent burns. **A = airway: no change. B = breathing: no change. C = compressions: no change. D = defibrillation: no change.**
Cardiac arrest and injury	**Assess scene and victim: no change. A = airway: change.** Clear mouth of blood, vomit, and other secretions. **B = breathing: no change. C = compressions: no change. D = defibrillation: no change.**

References

1. American Heart Association. Part 4: Adult basic life support. *Circulation* 2005; 112;IV-18-1V-34.

2. Madl C, Holzer M. Brain function after resuscitation from cardiac arrest. *Curr Opin Crit Care.* 2004 June; 10(3):213-7.

3. Mejicano GC, Maki DG. Infections acquired during cardiopulmonary resuscitation: Estimating the risk and defining strategies for prevention. *Ann Intern Med* 1998 November 15; 129(10):813-28.

4. U.S. Department of Health and Human Services, Centers for Disease Control and Prevention National Center for Chronic Disease Prevention and Health Promotion. Preventing heart disease and stroke: Addressing the nation's leading killers. www.cdc.gov/nccdphp/aag/aag_cvd.htm. Accessed 2006 August.

5. Statistics Canada. Selected leading causes of death, by sex (1997). www40.statcan.ca/l01/cst01/health36.htm?sdi=causes%20death. Accessed 2006 September.

6. World Health Organization. The atlas of heart disease and stroke. www.who.int/cardiovascular_diseases/resources/atlas/en. Accessed 2006 August.

7. U.S. Department of Health and Human Services, Centers for Disease Control and Prevention National Center for Chronic Disease Prevention and Health Promotion. Preventing heart disease and stroke: Addressing the nation's leading killers. www.cdc.gov/nccdphp/aag/aag_cvd.htm. Accessed 2006 August.

8. U.S. Department of Health and Human Services, Centers for Disease Control and Prevention National Center for Chronic Disease Prevention and Health Promotion. Preventing heart disease and stroke: Addressing the nation's leading killers. www.cdc.gov/nccdphp/aag/aag_cvd.htm. Accessed 2006 August.

9. U.S. Department of Labor Occupational Safety & Health Administration. Cardiac arrest and automated external defibrillators (AEDs). Recommendations. Technical information bulletin. www.osha.gov/dts/tib/tib_data/tib20011217.html. Accessed August 2006.

10. National Heart, Lung, and Blood Institute (NHLBI). How can I prevent a heart attack? www.nhlbi.nih.gov/health/dci/Diseases/HeartAttack/HeartAttack_Prevention.html. Accessed 2006 August.

11. Merck & Co. The Merck manual of diagnoses and therapy. Section 16. Cardiovascular disorders, chapter 202: Coronary artery disease. www.merck.com/mrkshared/mmanual/section16/chapter202/202a.jsp. Accessed 2006 August.

12. Antman EM, et al. ACC/AHA guidelines for the management of victims with ST-elevation myocardial infarction. A report of the American College of Cardiology/American Heart Association Task Force on Practice Guidelines (Committee to revise the 1999 guidelines for the Management of Acute Myocardial Infarction). http://guidelines.gov/summary/summary.aspx?doc_id=5457&nbr=3734. Accessed 2006 September.

13. National Institute of Neurological Disorders and Stroke, National Institutes of Health. August 7, 2006. NINDS stroke information page. www.ninds.nih.gov/disorders/stroke/stroke.htm. Accessed 2006 August.

14. Liferidge AT, Brice JH, Overby BA, Evenson KR. Ability of laypersons to use the Cincinnati Prehospital Stroke Scale. *Prehosp Emerg Care* 2004 October-December; 8(4):384-7.

15. American Heart Association. 2006. Learn to recognize a stroke. www.strokeassociation.org/presenter.jhtml?identifier=1020. Accessed 2006 August.

16. The Heart Rhythm Foundation. Sudden cardiac arrest key facts. www.heartrhythmfoundation.org/facts/scd.asp. Accessed 2006 September.

17. Medline Plus. Ventricular fibrillation. www.nlm.nih.gov/medlineplus/print/ency/article/007200.htm. Accessed 19 October 2005.

18. Heart Rhythm Society. Sudden cardiac death. www.hrspatients.org/patients/heart_disorders/cardiac_arrest/default.asp. Accessed 2006 August.

19. Newman MM. The chain of survival takes hold. *JEMS* 1989; 14 (8):11-13.

20. Hau SR, et al. Factors impeding dispatcher-assisted telephone cardiopulmonary resuscitation. *Ann Emerg Med* 2003 December; 42(6):731-7.

21. Roppolo LP, et al. Council of Standards Pre-Arrival Instruction Committee, National Academies of Emergency Dispatch modified cardiopulmonary resuscitation (CPR) instruction protocols for emergency medical dispatchers: Rationale and recommendations. *Resuscitation* 2005 May; 65(2):203-10.

22. Reed DB, et al. Location of cardiac arrests in the public access defibrillation trial. *Prehosp Emerg Care* 2006 January-March; 10(1):61-76.

23. Heart and Stroke Foundation of Canada. Chain of survival. http://ww1.heartandstroke.bc.ca/page.asp?PageID=388&LetterCode=67#Chain%20of%20survival. Accessed 2006 September.

24. Safe Kids Worldwide. Safety tips. www.safekids.org/tips/tips.html. Accessed 2006 August.

25. Thompson DC, Rivara FP. Pool fencing for preventing drowning in children. *Cochrane Database of Systematic Reviews* 1998; 1: CD001047. DOI: 10.1002/14651858.CD001047.

26. National Institute of Child Health and Human Development (NICHD). November 2005. SIDS: "Back to sleep" campaign. www.nichd.nih.gov/sids. Accessed 2006 August.

27. Hauck FR, Omojokun OO, Siadaty MS. Do pacifiers reduce the risk of sudden infant death syndrome? A meta-analysis. *Pediatrics* 2005 November; 116(5):e716-23.

28. Lopez-Herce J, et al. Long-term outcome of paediatric cardiorespiratory arrest in Spain. *Resuscitation* 2005 January; 64(1):79-85.

29. American Heart Association. 2006. *BLS for health care providers student manual.* Dallas, TX: American Heart Association.

30. Rathgeber J, et al. Influence of different types of recovery positions on perfusion indices of the forearm. *Resuscitation* 1996 July; 32(1):13-7.

31. Mejicano GC, Maki DG. Infections acquired during cardiopulmonary resuscitation: Estimating the risk and defining strategies for prevention. *Ann Intern Med* 1998 November 15; 129(10):813-28.

32. Wenzel V, Idris AH, Banner MJ, Fuerst RS, Tucker KJ. The composition of gas given by mouth-to-mouth ventilation during CPR. *Chest* 1994 December; 106(6):1806-10.

33. Koksal N, Buyukbese MA, Guven A, Cetinkaya A, Hasanoglu HC. Organophosphate intoxication as a consequence of mouth-to-mouth breathing from an affected case. *Chest* 2002 August; 122(2):740-1.

34. U.S. Food and Drug Administration. December 31, 2004. Section 503(b)(4) of the Food, Drug, and Cosmetic Act; 21 CFR Sections 201.(b)(1) and 211.130. www.fda.gov/opacom/laws/fdcact/fdctoc.htm. Accessed 2006 August.

35. Ewy GA. Cardiocerebral resuscitation: The new cardiopulmonary resuscitation. *Circulation* 2005 April 26; 111(16):2134-42.

36. Valenzuela TD, et al. Interruptions of chest compressions during emergency medical systems resuscitation. *Circulation* 2005 August 30; 112(9):1259-65.

37. Kern KB, et al. Importance of continuous chest compressions during cardiopulmonary resuscitation: Improved outcome during a simulated single lay-rescuer scenario. *Circulation* 2002 February 5; 105(5):645-9.

38. Hoke RS, Chamberlain D. Skeletal chest injuries secondary to cardiopulmonary resuscitation. *Resuscitation* 2004 December; 63(3):327-38.

39. Valenzuela TD, Roe DJ, Nichol G, Clark LL, Spaite DW, Hardman RG. Outcomes of rapid defibrillation by security officers after cardiac arrest in casinos. *N Engl J Med* 2000 October 26; 343(17):1206-9.

40. Samson RA, et al. Use of automated external defibrillators for children: An update. Advisory statement from the pediatric advanced life support task force, International Liaison Committee on Resuscitation. *Circulation* 2003 July 1; 107(25):3250-5.

41. Atkins DL, Jorgenson DB. Attenuated pediatric electrode pads for automated external defibrillator use in children. *Resuscitation* 2005 July; 66(1):31-7.

42. Ganz, L. October 8, 2004. Implantable cardioverter/defibrillators. www.emedicine.com/med/topic3386.htm. Accessed 2006 August.

43. ECRI (formerly the Emergency Care Research Institute), Medical Devices Safety Reports. 2006. Fires from defibrillation during oxygen administration hazard. *Health Devices* July 1994; 23(7):307-8. www.mdsr.ecri.org/summary/detail.aspx?doc_id=8128. Accessed 2006 August.

44. Robertshaw H, McAnulty G. Ambient oxygen concentrations during simulated cardiopulmonary resuscitation. *Anaesthesia* 1998 July; 53(7):634-7.

45. Monsieurs KG, Vogels C, Bossaert LL, Meert P, Calle PA. A study comparing the usability of fully automatic versus semi-automatic defibrillation by untrained nursing students. *Resuscitation* 2005 January; 64(1): 41-7.

46. Sandroni C, et al. Automated external defibrillation by untrained deaf lay rescuers. *Resuscitation* 2004 October; 63(1): 43-8.

47. Wik L, Dorph E, Auestad B, Steen PA. Evaluation of a defibrillator-basic cardiopulmonary resuscitation programme for non medical personnel. *Resuscitation* 2003 February; 56(2): 167-72.

48. Gundry JW, Comess KA, DeRook FA, Jorgenson D, Bardy GH. Comparison of naive sixth-grade children with trained professionals in the use of an automated external defibrillator. *Circulation* 1999 October 19; 100(16):1703-7.

49. Callejas S, Barry A, Demertsidis E, Jorgenson D, Becker LB. Human factors impact successful lay person automated external defibrillator use during simulated cardiac arrest. *Crit Care Med* 2004 September; 32(9 Suppl):S406-13.

50. Beckers S, et al. Minimal instructions improve the performance of laypersons in the use of semi-automatic and automatic external defibrillators. *Crit Care* 2005 April; 9(2):R110-6.

51. Pagan-Carlo LA, Spencer KT, Robertson CE, Dengler A, Birkett C, Kerber RE. Transthoracic defibrillation: Importance of avoiding electrode placement directly on the female breast. *J Am Coll Cardiol* 1996; 27:449-452.

52. Macdonald RD, Swanson JM, Mottley JL, Weinstein C. Performance and error analysis of automated external defibrillator use in the out-of-hospital setting. *Ann Emerg Med* 2001 September; 38(3):262-7.

53. Ko PC, Lin CH, Lu TC, Ma MH, Chen WJ, Lin FY. Machine and operator performance analysis of automated external defibrillator utilization. *J Formos Med Assoc* 2005 July; 104(7):476-81.

54. U.S. Department of Health and Human Services, Centers for Disease Control and Prevention. Non-fatal choking-related episodes for children 0 to 14 years of age—United States, 2001. *MMWR (Morbidity and Mortality Weekly Report)* 2002.

55. Chiu CY, Wong KS, Lai SH, Hsia SH, Wu CT. Factors predicting early diagnosis of foreign body aspiration in children. *Pediatr Emerg Care* 2005 March; 21(3):161-4.

56. Morley RE, et al. Foreign body aspiration in infants and toddlers: recent trends in British Columbia. *J Otolaryngol.* 2004 February; 33(1):37-41.

57. Berzlanovich AM. Foreign body asphyxia: A preventable cause of death in the elderly. *Am J Prev Med* 2005 January; 28(1):65-9.

58. 2005 International Liaison Committee on Resuscitation, American Heart Association, European Resuscitation Council. Attitude toward performing CPR. 2005 International Consensus Conference on Cardiopulmonary Resuscitation and Emergency Cardiovascular Care Science with Treatment Recommendations. Dallas, TX, January 23-30, 2005. *Circulation* 2005; 112:III-100-III-108 and *Resuscitation* 2005 December; 67(1): S1-S190.

59. Shenefelt, R. Emotional aspects of basic life support. Presentation of Scientific Program of the New Zealand Resuscitation Council Conference, Wellington, NZ. November 1999.

60. Morgan R, Westmoreland C. Survey of junior hospital doctors' attitudes to cardiopulmonary resuscitation. *Postgrad Med J* 2002 July; 78(921):413-5.

61. Gamble M. A debriefing approach to dealing with the stress of CPR attempts. *Prof Nurse* 2001 November; 17(3):157-60.

62. Axelsson A, et al. Factors surrounding cardiopulmonary resuscitation influencing bystanders' psychological reactions. *Resuscitation* 1998 April; 37(1):13-20.

63. Swanson RW. Psychological issues in CPR. *Ann Emerg Med* 1993 February; 22(2 Pt 2):350-3.

64. Newman M. CPR comes full circle. *J Emerg Med Serv* 1990; 15(4):48-55.

65. Lederer W, Mair D, Rabl W, Baubin M. Frequency of rib and sternum fractures associated with out-of-hospital cardiopulmonary resuscitation is underestimated by conventional chest X-ray. *Resuscitation* 2004 February; 60(2):157-62.

66. Hoke RS, Chamberlain D. Skeletal chest injuries secondary to cardiopulmonary resuscitation. *Resuscitation* 2004 December; 63(3):327-38.

67. American Heart Association. Guidelines for cardiopulmonary resuscitation (CPR) and emergency cardiovascular care (ECC). Part 2: Ethical issues. *Circulation* 2005; 112.

68. Bangor Hydro Electric Company. First responder safety. www.bhe.com/safety/responder.cfm. Accessed 2006 August.

CPR and AED for Professionals

Note to readers: The procedures described in this chapter are intended **only** for health care providers, first responders, and professional rescuers either in a hospital or in other settings and for those needing professional-level basic life support training as a job requirement. If you are learning CPR in order to help others in the community or in your workplace on a volunteer basis, you should read chapter 3. American Safety & Health Institute (ASHI) certification may be issued only when an ASHI-authorized instructor verifies you have successfully completed and competently performed the required core knowledge and skill objectives of the program. By itself, this chapter does not constitute complete training.

Because the audience for Human Kinetics' courses is nonmedical professional rescuers, we have used the term "victim" instead of the typical medically-oriented term "patient."

In this book, the term *basic life support* (BLS) means recognizing signs of sudden cardiac arrest (SCA), heart attack, stroke, and foreign-body airway obstruction (FBAO); administering cardiopulmonary resuscitation (CPR); and using an automated external defibrillator (AED),[1] when appropriate.

The basic life support procedures and skills you will learn in this chapter include the following:

- How the respiratory and circulatory systems work
- How to identify types of heart disease and stroke and provide first aid for them
- How to follow the emergency action steps for adults, children, and infants:

    - Rescue breathing
    - Chest compressions
    - Using an AED

- How to aid adults, children, and infants who are choking
- Key psychological and legal aspects of providing basic life support
- How to alter the standard emergency action steps to accommodate special conditions

Figure 4.1 shows the basic life support procedures to be taught in this chapter.

When you provide BLS, you help the victim's respiratory and circulatory systems to function. The next two sections provide brief descriptions of how these systems work.

Universal Basic Life Support Procedures*

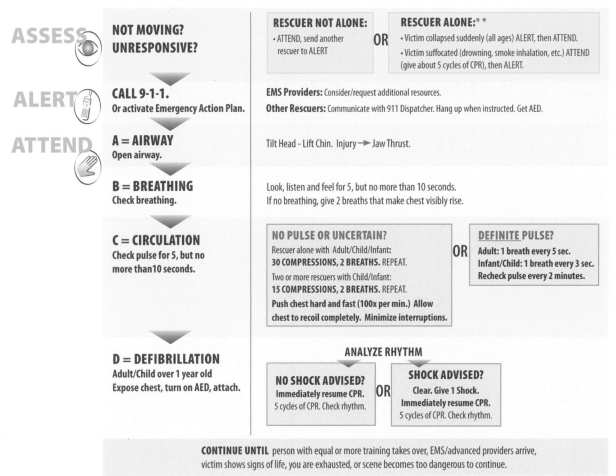

ASSESS

NOT MOVING?
UNRESPONSIVE?

RESCUER NOT ALONE:
• ATTEND, send another rescuer to ALERT

OR

RESCUER ALONE:*
• Victim collapsed suddenly (all ages) ALERT, then ATTEND.
• Victim suffocated (drowning, smoke inhalation, etc.) ATTEND (give about 5 cycles of CPR), then ALERT.

ALERT

CALL 9-1-1.
Or activate Emergency Action Plan.

EMS Providers: Consider/request additional resources.

Other Rescuers: Communicate with 911 Dispatcher. Hang up when instructed. Get AED.

ATTEND

A = AIRWAY
Open airway.

Tilt Head - Lift Chin. Injury ➔ Jaw Thrust.

B = BREATHING
Check breathing.

Look, listen and feel for 5, but no more than 10 seconds.
If no breathing, give 2 breaths that make chest visibly rise.

C = CIRCULATION
Check pulse for 5, but no more than 10 seconds.

NO PULSE OR UNCERTAIN?
Rescuer alone with Adult/Child/Infant:
30 COMPRESSIONS, 2 BREATHS. REPEAT.
Two or more rescuers with Child/Infant:
15 COMPRESSIONS, 2 BREATHS. REPEAT.
Push chest hard and fast (100x per min.) Allow chest to recoil completely. Minimize interruptions.

OR

DEFINITE PULSE?
Adult: 1 breath every 5 sec.
Infant/Child: 1 breath every 3 sec.
Recheck pulse every 2 minutes.

D = DEFIBRILLATION
Adult/Child over 1 year old
Expose chest, turn on AED, attach.

ANALYZE RHYTHM

NO SHOCK ADVISED?
Immediately resume CPR.
5 cycles of CPR. Check rhythm.

OR

SHOCK ADVISED?
Clear. Give 1 Shock.
Immediately resume CPR.
5 cycles of CPR. Check rhythm.

CONTINUE UNTIL person with equal or more training takes over, EMS/advanced providers arrive, victim shows signs of life, you are exhausted, or scene becomes too dangerous to continue.

*Procedure adapted from *Circulation* 2005; 112: III-3, IV-21, IV-158 © 2005 International Liaison Committee on Resuscitation, American Heart Association,® Inc. and European Resuscitation Council.
** Sudden collapse more likely caused by VF, requiring early defibrillation. Suffocation more likely to respond to early CPR.

Figure 4.1   Universal basic life support procedures.

Respiratory System

Each cell of the body requires a regular supply of oxygen in order to stay alive. Because the body cannot store oxygen, as it does with food and water, we must continually breathe oxygen into the lungs. Respiration is taking in oxygen and giving off carbon dioxide. The respiratory system is a collection of organs involved in this process. The system, shown in figure 4.2, is made up of *(a)* the lungs, *(b)* bronchial tubes, *(c)* nose, *(d)* mouth, *(e)* windpipe, and *(f)* diaphragm. When you take a breath, the diaphragm moves down and the chest moves out, drawing air into the lungs. This

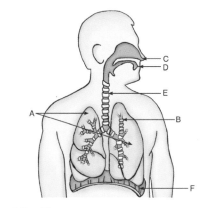

Figure 4.2   The respiratory system.

is called *inhalation*. The air we inhale contains approximately 21% oxygen. In the lungs, oxygen is absorbed into the bloodstream and circulated throughout the body. When the diaphragm moves up, air exits the lungs in *exhalation*. Carbon dioxide is released in the exhaled air. Not all of the oxygen is used by the body in the breathing process. Exhaled air contains about 16 to 17% oxygen. When delivered during rescue breathing, this is enough oxygen to support life.

Circulatory System

The circulatory system uses the bloodstream to deliver oxygen and nutrients to body tissues and removes waste products from them. Figure 4.3 is a simplified drawing of the circulatory system. The driving force of the system is the heart *(a)*. Special tissue runs throughout the heart that is capable of creating and conducting electric current. This electric current triggers the rhythmic mechanical contractions that create a flow of blood through the body's blood vessels and heart, which is known as circulation. Large vessels called arteries *(b)* carry oxygenated blood from the heart to body tissues. Capillaries *(c)* are where oxygen, nutrients, and waste products are exchanged and where arteries connect to veins *(d)* to return used blood back to the heart. From there, the used blood is sent to the lungs, where carbon dioxide is released and fresh oxygen is picked up. The fresh blood is returned to the heart, and the cycle repeats.

The body cannot survive when circulation stops. Brain tissue is especially sensitive to a lack of oxygen. External chest compressions combined with rescue breathing (CPR) are essential for providing blood flow to vital organs during cardiac arrest. Immediate CPR can double or triple a victim's chance of survival. Unfortunately, the majority of cardiac arrest survivors remain in a coma for varying lengths of time, and full brain recovery is rare.[2]

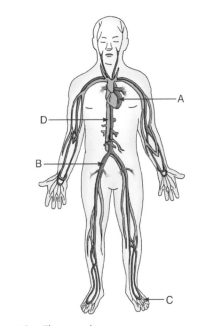

Figure 4.3   The circulatory system.

Universal Precautions

As described in chapter 1, universal precautions are a way to limit the spread of disease by preventing rescuers from having contact with blood and body fluids. To observe universal precautions means that whether or not you think the victim's blood or body fluid is infected, you act as if it is.

The risk of contracting a disease while giving BLS is extremely low. No documented cases exist of human immunodeficiency virus (HIV), hepatitis B (HBV), or hepatitis C (HCV) infection transmitted by mouth-to-mouth ventilation. The estimated risk for acquiring HIV, HBV, or HCV infection during basic life support is extremely low—about one in one million. There have been no reports of infection acquired during CPR training. Simple infection-control measures, including use of barrier devices, can reduce the risk for acquisition of an infectious disease during CPR and CPR training.[3]

While the risk of disease is low when you perform CPR, observing universal precautions with victims of all ages will make it lower. Using face shields (see figure 4.4) and masks allows you to perform rescue breathing and reduce the risk of compromising your own health. These devices are usually available for all ages and sizes. They come with a replaceable one-way valve or filters to block contaminated fluids.

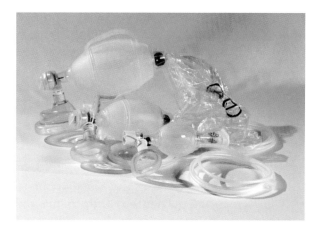

Figure 4.5   Bag-mask devices.

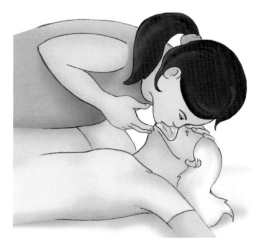

Figure 4.4   Rescue breathing with a face shield.

One problem with face shields is that they do not prevent contamination of the rescuer's side of the shield. Thus, to reduce the risk of transmitting infection as a professional rescuer, you should use a face shield only as an emergency substitute for mouth-to-mouth breathing and switch to a mask or bag-mask device (see figure 4.5) as soon as possible.

Bag-mask devices are used in various clinical and emergency settings to provide oxygen and ventilation to a victim who is not breathing or is not breathing adequately. When used with supplemental oxygen, the bag-mask device can provide up to 100% oxygen on every squeeze and release of the bag. Health care providers, first responders, and professional rescuers should have these devices available in adult sizes and several pediatric sizes. Training is needed for safe and effective use of the bag-mask device.

Be sure to wear other types of personal protective equipment as necessary, such as gloves and goggles. Follow the procedures that you learned in chapter 1 for preventing infection from pathogens.

Heart Disease and Stroke

Heart disease and stroke—the main components of cardiovascular disease—are the leading causes of death for both men and women in the United States and account for nearly 40% of all deaths.[4] More than 927,000 Americans die of cardiovascular disease each year, which amounts to 1 death every 34 seconds. Heart disease and stroke are also the main causes of adult deaths in Canada.[5] By 2020 heart disease and stroke will become the leading cause of both death and disability worldwide; the number of deaths is projected to increase to more than 20 million a year.[6]

The major independent risk factors for heart disease and stroke are high blood pressure and high blood cholesterol. A 12- to 13-point reduction in blood pressure can reduce heart attacks by 21%, strokes by 37%, and all deaths from cardiovascular disease by 25%.[4]

Everyone should know the signs and symptoms of heart attack and stroke and the impor-

Lowering Your Risk for Cardiovascular Disease

You can lower your risk for cardiovascular disease by making healthy lifestyle choices such as these:

- Eat a healthy diet to prevent or reduce high blood pressure and high blood cholesterol. A healthy diet is high in fruits and vegetables, whole grains, and lean protein and low in saturated fat, cholesterol, trans fat, artificial preservatives, refined carbohydrate, and sugar.
- Maintain a healthy weight.
- Control your alcohol intake.
- Don't smoke.
- Exercise as directed by your doctor.
- Lose weight if you are overweight or obese.[7, 8]

tance of calling 9-1-1 quickly; almost half (47%) of heart attack victims and about the same percentage of stroke victims die before EMS personnel arrive.[4] Family members of victims who have had a recent heart attack should take CPR training and be familiar with the use of an automated external defibrillator (AED, described on page 105). All health care providers, first responders, and professional rescuers who respond to victims with chest pain and suspected cardiac arrest should be equipped with and trained in the use of AEDs.

The next sections cover the signs and symptoms and treatment guidelines for acute coronary syndrome, stroke, and sudden cardiac arrest.

Acute Coronary Syndrome

The major complication of cardiovascular disease is *acute coronary syndrome* (ACS). This term applies to several conditions and symptoms ranging from unstable angina to myocardial infarction (heart attack). ACS occurs when the heart does not get enough oxygenated blood flow. If the blood flow to the heart is cut off, a part of the heart will die, causing disability or death. Figure 4.6 shows damage to heart muscle from inadequate blood supply. ACS is the cause of sudden cardiac arrest in most adult victims.

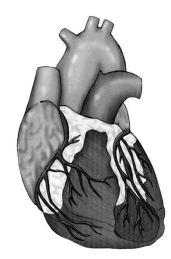

Figure 4.6 Damage to heart muscle.

Signs and Symptoms

There is a wide range, from slight to severe:

- Chest pain or a dull discomfort behind the breastbone that may or may not spread to the arms, back, neck, jaw, or stomach
- Shortness of breath
- Weakness, nausea, dizziness
- Heavy sweating
- Fear of impending doom (feeling like something extremely bad is going to happen but not sure what)

CAUTION!

The absence of chest pain, especially in people with diabetes, women, and the elderly, does not mean that the victim is not at risk. Unusual symptoms of heart attack include headache, ringing in the ears, dizziness, hiccups, and belching. **Do not** downplay the seriousness of the potential problem.

- Uncertainty and embarrassment
- Denial (victim often refuses to accept or believe he or she may be having a heart attack, which can delay treatment and increase the risk of death)

Treatment Guidelines

1. Place the victim in a comfortable position.
2. Assist with administration of the victim's own prescribed nitroglycerin (placed or sprayed under the tongue). If chest discomfort or pain does not improve or worsens, repeat the dosage of nitroglycerin according to the doctor's orders.
3. If the victim does not have a history of aspirin allergy, advise the victim to chew and swallow a half or whole adult tablet (162 to 325 milligrams) of aspirin.
4 Administer supplementary oxygen.
5. Comfort, calm, and reassure the victim.

Stroke

A *stroke* happens when the blood supply to part of the brain is suddenly interrupted or when a blood vessel in the brain bursts, spilling blood into the spaces surrounding brain cells. Brain cells die when they no longer receive oxygen and nutrients from the blood or there is sudden bleeding into or around the brain (see figure 4.7).[9] Limiting the extent of brain damage caused by a stroke depends on rapid diagnosis and treatment in the hospital. This requires the victim, family members, or bystanders to quickly recognize the signs and symptoms of stroke and activate EMS.[10] To reduce brain injury and ensure the best recovery, EMS must be rapidly dispatched, you must quickly identify the potential stroke victim, and you must rapidly notify and transport the victim to a designated stroke center, if available.

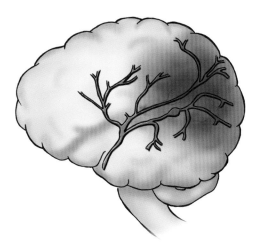

Figure 4.7   Damage to brain from stroke.

Risk factors for stroke include the following:

- High blood pressure
- Diabetes
- Smoking
- High cholesterol level
- Heart disease

Signs and Symptoms[11]

- *Sudden* numbness or weakness of the face, arm, or leg, especially on one side of the body
- *Sudden* confusion, trouble speaking, or trouble understanding
- *Sudden* trouble seeing in one or both eyes
- *Sudden* trouble walking, dizziness, loss of balance, or loss of coordination
- *Sudden*, severe headache
- Ministroke (transient ischemic attack, or TIA): same symptoms as a stroke, but it lasts for only a few minutes and may lead to stroke

Note: Victims of stroke are sometimes mistaken for being drunk.

CAUTION!

Stroke treatments are time sensitive!

Treatment Guidelines

If you suspect a stroke, ask the victim to do the following:

1. Smile
2. Raise both arms
3. Speak a simple sentence

If the victim has any trouble with these three tasks, he or she may be having a stroke. Alert EMS or activate your emergency action plan immediately. You should administer supplementary oxygen as trained or according to doctor's orders. Also comfort, calm, and reassure the victim.

Sudden Cardiac Arrest

Sudden cardiac arrest (SCA) occurs when the heart's electrical system malfunctions and the heart abruptly stops working without warning. SCA is one of the leading causes of death among adults in North America.[12] When SCA occurs, most victims have an abnormal heart rhythm known as *ventricular fibrillation* (VF). The most common cause of VF is a poor supply of oxygen to the heart, most commonly caused by heart attack.[13] After a heart attack, low oxygen can cause the heart's natural electronic signals to become disorganized. This causes twitching of the heart muscle (VF) and prevents coordinated contraction. The heart stops pumping blood and oxygen to itself and to the brain. The lack of blood flow and oxygen supply to the brain causes the victim to lose consciousness immediately. Unless a shock is delivered to the heart to restore its regular rhythm, brain death can occur within minutes.

SCA often occurs in active, outwardly healthy people with no known heart disease or other health problems, but most victims have heart diseases or other health problems (although they may not know it). The most important risk factors are a previous heart attack and coronary artery disease (CAD, narrowed or blocked arteries supplying blood to the heart).[14]

An automated external defibrillator (AED) is a small, portable computerized device that diagnoses and treats VF (see figure 4.8). It is attached with wires and pads to the chest of the victim. It checks the person's heart rhythm, decides if the rhythm is VF, and gives the heart an electric shock. If this shock is delivered promptly after collapse, many victims can survive without brain damage. If an AED is available, immediately attach it to the victim. Listen and follow the machine's instructions.

Signs and Symptoms

- Sudden collapse without warning (some people may have a racing heartbeat or feel dizzy or faint)
- Unconsciousness or unresponsiveness
- Abnormal grunting, gasping, or snoring noises
- Looks dead

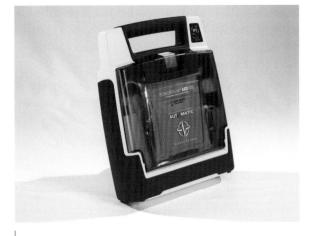

Figure 4.8   LIFEPAK CR Plus AED.
Courtesy Cardiac Science Corporation.

Sudden cardiac arrest should be treated with CPR and defibrillation using an AED as soon as possible.

Chain of Survival in Adults

The *chain of survival* is a concept used to communicate the key factors that must be in place if a victim is to survive sudden cardiac arrest (SCA) from ventricular fibrillation.[15] The links in the chain of survival include early identification of SCA, early CPR, early defibrillation, and early advanced life support (ALS). See figure 4.9.

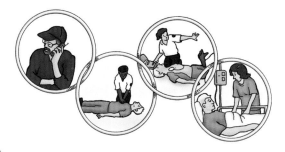

Figure 4.9   Chain of survival (adults).

- **Early identification.** The faster SCA is identified and the response system is activated, the better the chances that the victim will survive. Dispatcher-assisted telephone CPR instruction can increase the proportion of SCA victims who receive CPR from bystanders. It also has been associated with improved survival.[16, 17]

- **Early CPR.** Victims in cardiac arrest need immediate CPR. CPR provides a small but vital amount of blood flow to the heart and brain. CPR increases the chances that a shock from an AED will allow the heart to start working effectively.

- **Early defibrillation.** No more than 3 minutes from collapse to defibrillation is necessary for achieving the highest survival rates.[18]

- **Early ALS.** Advanced life support involves medical procedures and medications used by paramedics, nurses, and doctors to manage a victim's vital signs and organ systems to increase the chances of survival and recovery.

If any one of these links is weak or missing, the result will be poor survival. Some organizations have added further links to the chain. These include making healthy choices that reduce the risk of heart attack, stroke, and injury and restoring the victim to the highest possible level of functional ability (early rehabilitation).[19]

Chain of Survival in Children

The chain of survival in children emphasizes prevention, basic CPR, early identification of an emergency with rapid activation of an emergency action plan (including EMS), and early pediatric advanced life support (see figure 4.10). Except for those with heart problems, a child's heart does not usually stop suddenly, as is often the case in adults. Rather, the heart slows and then stops only after the child has not been breathing for an extended time. Breathing stops because of a lack of oxygen in the blood. This can be caused by respiratory diseases (such as asthma), injuries, and conditions such as drowning and sudden infant death syndrome (SIDS).

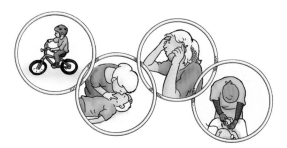

Figure 4.10   Chain of survival (children).

When an infant or child stops breathing but his or her heart continues to beat and rescue breathing is quickly provided, survival with normal (or near-normal) brain function is much higher, reportedly as much as 70%.[24] Giving infants and children rescue breaths that make the chest visibly rise is very important. When a rescuer finds a child unresponsive and not moving, he or she should give 2 minutes of CPR before calling 9-1-1 or attaching an AED. If another rescuer is present, he or she should activate the EMS or emergency action plan.

Prevention

- **Injuries.** Injury is a leading killer of children 14 and under worldwide. Most injuries can be prevented by the use of simple safety measures.[20]
- **Drowning.** Death rates are highest in children less than 5 years of age. Pool fencing significantly reduces the risk of drowning. Pool fences with a secure, self-latching gate should be installed around all public, semipublic, and private pools.[21]
- **SIDS.** Placing infants on their backs to sleep and giving them a pacifier significantly reduces the risk of sudden infant death syndrome (SIDS).[22, 23]

Emergency Action Steps

EMERGENCY ACTION STEPS

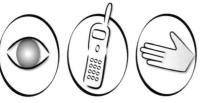

Assess – Alert – Attend to the ABCDs

The emergency action steps are **assess, alert,** and **attend to the ABCDs.** They are intended to help you, as a rescuer, respond to an emergency and manage life-threatening problems of the airway, breathing, and circulation of an adult, child, or infant. CPR procedures differ for adults, children, and infants. While no single factor can distinguish an infant from a child and a child from an adult, in order to simplify training, CPR guidelines use the age ranges in the following list:

Age Ranges for Adults, Children, and Infants

Adult = About onset of puberty

Child = About 1 year to onset of puberty

Infant = Less than about 1 year

Newborn = Birth until baby leaves hospital

Note the use of the word *about* in the previous list. When it comes to basic life support, determining age can be difficult. Exactness is not necessary.

The following text contains integrated recommendations for adults, children, and infants. For quick reference, refer to the Skill Guides on pages 118 to 125.

Assess

Assess the scene, then assess the victim.

- **Assess the scene.** Assess for safety. If the scene is not safe or at any time becomes unsafe, **get out!** See figure 4.11.

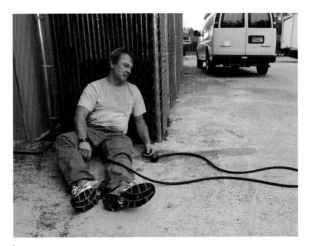

Figure 4.11 Unsafe scene.

- **Assess the victim.** If the scene is safe, pause for a moment as you approach the victim. What is your first impression? Is the victim lying still or moving around? Does skin color appear normal for the victim's ethnic group? Does it look difficult for the victim to breathe? Normal breathing is quiet and easy. Signs that basic life support or CPR may be needed include the following:

- Victim is not moving, is unresponsive, or looks dead.
- Skin tissue is bluish or ashen, especially around the lips.
- Skin tissue is cold and pale.
- Breathing is shallow, gasping, or absent.
- Pink or frothy discharge from mouth is present.

Gently tap or squeeze the victim's shoulder and ask, "Are you all right?" For an infant, you may tap the foot. Use the victim's name if you know it.

Alert

If the victim responds but is badly hurt, looks or acts very ill, or quickly gets worse, alert EMS (if you are in the United States or Canada call 9-1-1) or activate your emergency action plan. Use the following guidelines when you are responding in these situations:

• **Rescuer alone.** If you are alone, you should modify your approach to the victim based on the most likely cause of the problem. If the victim collapsed suddenly (all ages), first shout for help and, if someone responds, send him or her to alert EMS or activate the emergency action plan and to get an AED (and oxygen when readily available). Then attend to the victim. If no one responds to your shout for help, alert EMS or activate the emergency action plan yourself, then quickly return to attend to the victim. Getting the AED as soon as possible is important because a sudden collapse in adults and children is almost always caused by sudden cardiac arrest and requires early defibrillation. On the other hand, if you discover an unresponsive victim who suffocated (such as from drowning, smoke inhalation, or some other cause), first attend to the victim. Give 5 cycles of CPR (about 2 minutes) before leaving to alert EMS or activate the emergency action plan and get the AED and oxygen. This is because a victim who suffocated is more likely to respond to early CPR due to the low oxygen levels in blood and tissues (hypoxia).

• **Rescuer not alone.** If more than one rescuer is present, procedures should occur simultaneously. One or more rescuers remain with the victim and begin the steps of CPR. Another alerts EMS or activates the emergency action plan and gets the AED and oxygen.

• **EMS providers.** If you are an EMS provider, when arriving on the scene of a potential cardiac arrest, always bring the appropriate equipment to the victim, including the AED, oxygen, and ventilation devices. After assessing the scene and forming a general impression of the victim, consider requesting additional personnel and resources.

Attend to the ABCDs

The ABCDs are the action steps you should take when attending to the victim: airway, breathing, circulation, and defibrillation. To properly attend to the victim, you must place him or her faceup on a firm, flat surface. If the victim is lying facedown, roll him or her over. Try to minimize turning or twisting of the head and neck.

A = Airway

The airway is the passageway between the mouth and lungs. It must be open so air can enter and leave the lungs freely. Blockage of the airway in an adult or child is commonly caused by the tongue. To open the airway, tilt the victim's head and lift the chin.

If you suspect a cervical spine injury, open the airway using a jaw thrust without the head tilt. Place one hand on each side of the victim's head. Then place your fingers under the angles of the victim's lower jaw and lift the jaw forward with both hands.

Because maintaining an open airway and providing adequate ventilation are a critical priority, if the jaw thrust does not open the airway, use the head tilt and chin lift maneuver (see figure 4.12). In an infant, chin lift and jaw thrust are proven methods for opening an obstructed upper airway.[25, 26]

B = Breathing

While keeping the airway open, look, listen, and feel for breathing for at least 5 seconds, but no longer than 10 seconds.[27] Opening the airway

CAUTION!

Don't use your thumb to open the airway or press too hard on the soft area under the chin. Doing so can block the airway. Also, don't push the mouth completely closed.

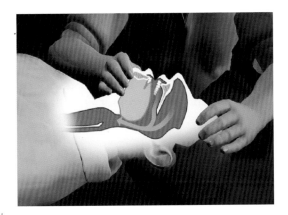

Figure 4.12 Tilt head, lift chin to open airway.

might allow the victim to start breathing adequately. If the victim is breathing adequately or starts breathing adequately at any time, consider placing him or her in the recovery position. In this position, there is less chance of obstruction by the tongue and secretions. Make sure the victim's body position is stable so he or she does not roll onto the face or back. Also make sure there is no pressure on the chest that could make it more difficult to breathe. To prevent blood flow in the lower arm from being impaired, turn the victim to the opposite side if he or she is in the recovery position for more than 30 minutes.[28] If the victim is injured, use a modified recovery position called the HAINES method (described in chapter 2).

It may be difficult to determine whether the victim is breathing adequately. **Occasional gasps are not normal and do not supply the victim with enough oxygen to sustain life.** If the chest does not rise and fall and no air is exhaled, or if the victim is making strange gasping, noisy, snorting, or gurgling sounds and you are not *positive* that the victim is breathing adequately, give two rescue breaths (ventilation without compression) immediately. Give each breath in 1 second and make the chest visibly rise. If the victim's chest does not rise with the first rescue breath,

reposition the head, make a better seal, and try again. **With children, you may have to try a couple of times to give two rescue breaths that make the chest visibly rise.** It is critical that rescue breaths make the infant or child's chest rise during rescue breathing and CPR.

Do not take deep breaths when performing rescue breathing. Taking deep breaths is unnecessary and may cause hyperventilation. If you suddenly feel breathless, have tiny prickling sensations, become dizzy, or have muscle spasms in your hands or feet, you are breathing too fast and deep. Slow down or have another rescuer take over for you.

Air is often blown into the stomach instead of the lungs during rescue breathing. This can cause the victim to vomit and can limit lung movement, reducing the effectiveness of rescue breathing. To reduce the risk of inflating the stomach, give each breath in 1 second. Give enough air to make the chest visibly rise, but no more than that. Allow the victim to exhale completely between breaths. If the victim vomits, turn the victim on his or her side (or use suction equipment when available) so he or she doesn't inhale the fluid.

When you perform rescue breathing, you should have a barrier such as a mask or face shield between you and the victim for protection against bloodborne pathogens. However, if necessary, you can provide mouth-to-mouth or mouth-to-nose breathing. You may at some time have to administer rescue breathing to someone who has a stoma (an opening at the front of the neck into the windpipe), and, when it is available, you may also need to administer supplemental oxygen.

Finally, you may need to use cricoid pressure (or the Sellick maneuver) to prevent an unconscious victim from aspirating foreign material into the lungs.

Rescue Breathing With a Face Shield

Tilt the victim's head and lift the chin. Place the face shield over the victim's mouth and nose.

Place your mouth on the face shield over the victim's mouth. Pinch the victim's nose either under or over the shield. Give two rescue breaths that make the chest visibly rise, but no more than that. See figure 4.13. Switch to a mask or bag-mask device as soon as possible.

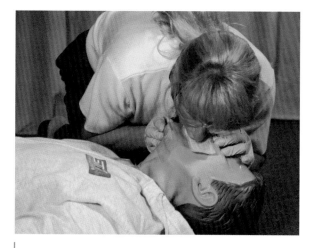

Figure 4.13 Rescue breathing with a face shield.

Rescue Breathing With a Mask

If you are alone, position yourself at the victim's side. Tilt the victim's head and lift the chin. Place the mask over the victim's mouth and nose. Place your mouth around the one-way valve on the mask and give two rescue breaths that make the chest visibly rise, but no more than that. See figure 4.14. Remove your mouth from the mask after each rescue breath and allow the victim to exhale. With an infant or small child, it is important to select a mask of the proper size.

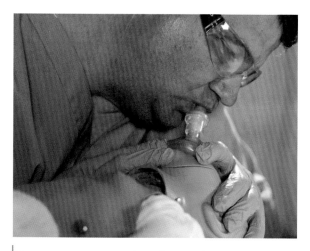

Figure 4.14 Rescue breathing with a mask.

Rescue Breathing With a Bag Mask

A bag mask is a device that has four main components: the bag, an oxygen reservoir, a one-way valve, and a mask. When used alone, the bag mask will allow delivery of 21% oxygen (room air) to the victim. This oxygen concentration is more than that delivered to a victim when you exhale during rescue breathing (17%). You can increase the amount of oxygen delivered with a bag mask by attaching an oxygen supply to the bag. When you use an oxygen source, attach a reservoir to the bag. The use of a bag mask with supplemental oxygen flowing at a rate of 15 liters per minute delivers approximately 100% oxygen to the victim.

When using a bag-mask device, open the victim's airway with a jaw lift and place the mask over the victim's mouth and nose. While keeping the airway open, hold the mask tightly against the victim's face and squeeze the bag. Give each breath in 1 second. Give enough air to make the chest visibly rise, but no more than that. With an infant or small child, it is important to select a bag-mask device of the proper size.

Although a single rescuer can use a bag mask effectively, it's better to have two rescuers when possible. When two rescuers use a bag mask, one holds the mask in place and maintains an open airway while the other squeezes the bag (see figure 4.15). If rescuers have difficulty with the bag mask, they should use mouth-to-mask rescue breathing.

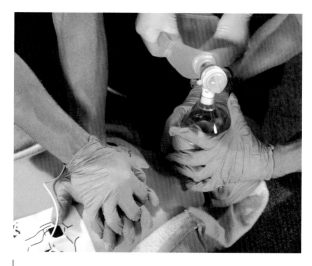

Figure 4.15 Rescue breathing with a bag-mask device during three-rescuer CPR.

CAUTION!

Ventilations are important for victims in cardiac arrest, but do not give too many breaths or breaths that are too large or too forceful. Excessive ventilation is unnecessary and harmful because it increases pressure in the victim's chest. This pressure decreases blood flow to and from the heart and reduces the already marginal flow of blood and oxygen during CPR, decreasing survival. **It is critical to avoid excessive ventilation.**

Advanced Airways

When professional rescuers are appropriately trained and authorized, they may use advanced airway and ventilation devices such as the laryngeal mask airway, Esophageal-Tracheal-Combitube, and endotracheal tube. When an advanced airway is in place, give rescue breaths at a rate of 1 breath every 6 to 8 seconds (8 to 10 breaths per minute). Do not pause chest compressions to ventilate.

Mouth-to-Mouth Rescue Breathing

A rescuer's exhaled air contains about 17% oxygen and 4% carbon dioxide.[29] This oxygen concentration is less than that delivered to the victim when using a bag-mask device without supplemental oxygen (21%), but it is enough to support life.

To provide mouth-to-mouth rescue breathing for an adult, child, or large infant (see the next section for instructions on performing mouth-to-nose rescue breathing on small infants), hold the victim's airway open, pinch the nose, and make a seal with your mouth over the victim's mouth. Give two breaths that make the chest visibly rise. Because of the risk of poisoning, do not perform mouth-to-mouth rescue breathing for victims who have been poisoned by phosphorus compounds, including insecticides and herbicides.[30]

Mouth-to-Nose Rescue Breathing

When you have difficulty with mouth-to-mouth rescue breathing, you may want to use mouth-to-nose rescue breathing. To give mouth-to-nose rescue breathing, tilt the victim's head back with one hand and use the other hand to close the victim's mouth. Seal your lips around the victim's nose and give slow breaths that make the chest rise. If the victim is an infant, place your mouth over the infant's mouth and nose.

Stoma

A stoma is a surgical opening at the front of the neck that extends into the windpipe. When an adult or child with a stoma requires rescue breathing, give mouth-to-stoma rescue breaths. See figure 4.16. As an option, you can cover the stoma with a child-sized face mask, place your mouth around the one-way valve on the mask, and give rescue breaths.

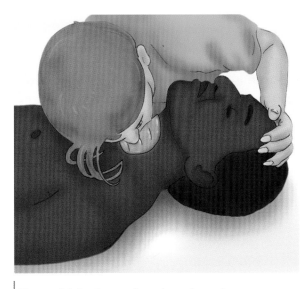

Figure 4.16   Rescue breathing through a stoma.

Supplemental Oxygen

Even the best chest compression provides only about 25 to 33% of the normal blood and oxygen flow from the heart. The combination of low blood flow and low oxygen causes organs to fail and leads to death. Giving rescue breathing with supplemental oxygen allows you to give rescue breaths with a higher concentration of oxygen. Oxygen-rich breaths deliver critically needed oxygen to the heart and brain. For this reason, when available, health care providers, first

Minimize Unprotected Rescue Breathing

Unprotected rescue breathing (mouth-to-mouth breathing) is a quick and effective way to provide oxygen to the victim. However, according to the U.S. Department of Labor, Occupational Safety & Health Administration (OSHA), unprotected mouth-to-mouth resuscitation should not be used by any emergency response personnel. Bag-valve masks and other equipment designed to isolate emergency response personnel from contact with the victim's saliva, respiratory secretions, vomit, blood, or body fluids should be available on all emergency vehicles and provided to all emergency response personnel who respond or potentially respond to medical emergencies or victim rescues.[31]

responders, and professional rescuers should use supplementary oxygen when performing rescue breathing. Ideally a bag-mask device should be attached to an oxygen reservoir to allow delivery of 100% oxygen to the victim.

Cricoid Pressure

Cricoid pressure (or the Sellick maneuver) is a means of preventing aspiration (inhaling stomach contents or foreign material into the lungs) in an unconscious victim. Aspiration is dangerous because it can cause acute respiratory failure, pneumonia, and airway obstruction.[32] Pressure is applied to the victim's cricoid cartilage. This pressure pushes the airway backward and squeezes the esophagus against the spine, preventing fluids or material from getting out of (and air from getting into) the stomach. To perform cricoid pressure, do the following:

1. Locate the thyroid cartilage (Adam's apple) with your index finger. The technique is often improperly applied. The safe and effective use requires knowledge of neck anatomy, proper training, and experience.

2. Slide your index finger downward to the bottom of the thyroid cartilage and feel for the indentation immediately below it. Just below the indentation is the cricoid cartilage (prominent horizontal ring).

3. Using the tips of your thumb and index finger, firmly press the cricoid cartilage directly backward (see figure 4.17). Do not push to one side or the other. If the victim gags, release the pressure.

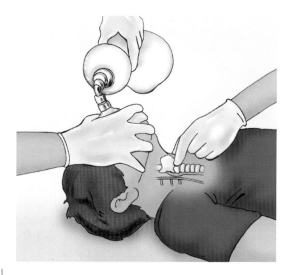

Figure 4.17   Applying cricoid pressure.

The technique is often improperly applied. The safe and effective use requires knowledge of neck anatomy, proper training, and experience.[33-35] It should be performed only by a trained and experienced rescuer and only when enough rescuers are present so there is no interruption in chest compressions or ventilations.

C = Circulation

For this step, begin by checking the victim's pulse to determine whether to administer only rescue breathing (ventilation without compression) or breathing and chest compressions. Different techniques are used for providing CPR to adults and children and to infants as well as when more than one rescuer is involved.

Check Pulse

If there is no response to the initial rescue breaths, feel for a pulse. Use the carotid pulse (neck) in adults, carotid or femoral (groin) in a child, and brachial (inside of the upper arm) in an infant. Studies show that health care providers, first responders, and professional rescuers take too long to check for a pulse and have difficulty determining whether a pulse is present or absent. For that reason, take at least 5, but no more than 10, seconds to check for a pulse. If you do not definitely feel a pulse, or if you are uncertain, immediately begin chest compressions, even if the victim is still taking occasional gasps. In a child, start chest compressions if the pulse is fewer than 60 beats per minute and there are signs of reduced blood flow such as poor color. (Count for 6 seconds and multiply by 10 to estimate heartbeats per minute. Do not count for a full minute.)

Note: Laypersons are taught not to check for a pulse before starting chest compressions.

Ventilation Without Compression

If the victim definitely has a pulse but is not breathing or not breathing adequately, provide ventilation without compression, also called rescue breathing.

• **For adults,** give 10 to 12 breaths per minute or about one breath every 5 to 6 seconds. Each breath should make the chest visibly rise. Reassess the pulse every couple of minutes for no more than 10 seconds.

• **For children and infants,** if the pulse is 60 beats per minute or more and the victim is not breathing or not breathing adequately, give rescue breaths, about 12 to 20 breaths per minute (1 breath every 3 to 5 seconds).

Note: Laypersons usually are not taught to provide rescue breathing without chest compressions.

External Chest Compressions

External chest compression is a rhythmic application of pressure over the breastbone. Chest compressions create blood flow to the heart, brain, and other organs by increasing pressure inside the chest and arteries and by direct com-

pression of the heart.[36] Creating and maintaining this pressure not only keep vital organs alive but also increase the chances that defibrillation will be successful.

Once chest compressions are started, it takes time to build up enough pressure to make blood flow. When chest compressions are stopped, the pressure and blood flow drop quickly. Thus, frequent interruption of chest compressions may contribute to poor survival rates.[37] For that reason, minimize interruptions in chest compressions during CPR.[38] Pause the chest compression as infrequently as possible. Limit interruptions to no longer than 10 seconds except when necessary to use a defibrillator or to perform advanced life support procedures such as intubation.

Compression techniques are different for infants than they are for adults and children. Be sure to use the following procedures:

• **Adults and children.** To make blood flow to the heart and brain effective, you must place the victim faceup and lying flat on a firm surface. Remove any clothing from the chest. Place the heel of one hand in the center of the chest between the nipples. See figure 4.18.

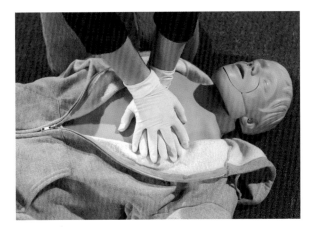

Figure 4.18 Adult: Push hard and fast.

Position yourself above the victim's chest so your shoulders are directly over your hands. Straighten your arms and lock your elbows. Put one hand on top of the other. Your fingers can be straight or fastened together, but you should keep them off the chest.

Use your upper-body weight to help compress the chest. **For a normal-sized adult,** push straight down on the chest approximately 1.5 to 2 inches (4 to 5 centimeters). **For a child,** use either one or two hands to compress the child's chest about one-third to one-half the depth of the chest (see figure 4.19). At the top of each compression, release pressure and completely remove your weight.

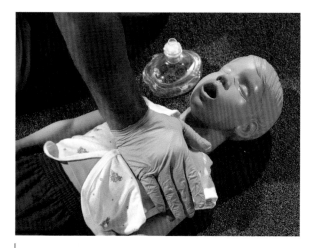

Figure 4.19   Child: Push hard and fast.

Chest compressions and relaxation should be about equal. Give 30 chest compressions at a speed of about 100 per minute. Keeping up the force, length, and speed of compressions helps create the best blood flow possible. Do not push over the lowest portion of the breastbone.

After 30 compressions, open the victim's airway and give two rescue breaths that make the chest visibly rise. Quickly resume chest compressions.

When adult chest compressions are given properly, you might hear an unpleasant sound like knuckles cracking. You might feel the breastbone fall in a bit. This is caused by cartilage or ribs cracking. Any damage done is not serious, so don't worry about it. Forceful external chest compression is critical if the victim is to survive without brain damage. In infants and toddlers, CPR rarely causes cracked ribs.[39]

•   **Infants.** If you are a single rescuer, compress the infant's breastbone with two fingertips placed just below the nipple line (see figure 4.20). You may place your other hand under the

infant's back to create a compression surface. Press down on the breastbone about one-third to one-half the depth of the infant's chest. After each compression, completely release the pressure on the breastbone and allow it to return to its normal position. Give 30 chest compressions at a speed of about 100 per minute.

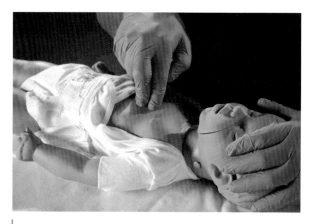

Figure 4.20   Infant: Push hard and fast.

When more than one rescuer is present, use two thumbs with your fingers encircling the chest and supporting the back for chest compression (see figure 4.21).

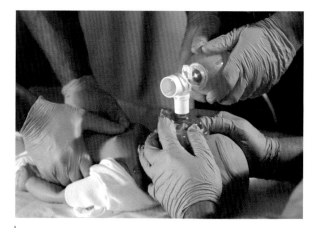

Figure 4.21   Two-thumb compression technique.

CPR With Two or More Rescuers

When more than one health care provider, first responder, or other professional rescuer are available to perform CPR, one gives chest compressions while the other keeps the airway open and performs rescue breathing. The rescuer compressing the chest should pause briefly to allow the two breaths to be given by the other rescuer. In children (up to the age of puberty) the ratio for compressions to breaths for two rescuers is 15:2 (3:1 for newborn infants). The ratio for adults is 30:2. However, once an advanced airway is inserted, the rescuer giving compressions should do so continuously, without pausing for ventilations. When an advanced airway is in place, give rescue breaths at a rate of 1 breath every 6 to 8 seconds (8 to 10 breaths per minute); this is the same for infants, children, and adults. Do not pause chest compressions to ventilate.

Studies have shown that rescuers quickly become tired while performing chest compressions. Compressions may become inadequate within as little as 1 minute.[40, 41] To prevent fatigue and maintain the quality of chest compressions, rescuers should change positions at least every couple of minutes. This should be done quickly, in less than 5 seconds, so there is as little interruption in compression as possible. AED rhythm checks should be very brief, and pulse checks should generally be performed only by an advanced life support provider).[42] If there is any doubt about the presence of a pulse, immediately resume chest compressions. Rescuers should continually monitor and encourage each other to perform good chest compression (hard and fast with complete recoil and minimal interruption).

D = Defibrillation

When sudden cardiac arrest occurs, most victims have an abnormal heart rhythm known as *ventricular fibrillation* (VF). If the heart can be shocked quickly with an AED, a normal heart rhythm may be restored. The following are some precautions that you must take before attaching the AED and the procedures for using the AED for adults and children. Defibrillation is not recommended for infants. Also presented are the steps to using an AED, troubleshooting and maintenance of the AED, and how the AED fits into an overall program of high-quality care.

Preparations Before AED Use

Before attaching the AED, quickly check for the following situations:

- **Chest hair.** If the victim's chest is covered with hair, it may prevent the electrode pads from making effective contact with the skin. If the AED voice prompt continues to say, "Check pads" or something similar after you attach the pads, quickly remove the pads, tearing out the hair under them. Apply a second set of electrodes. If the problem continues, quickly shave the chest in the area of the pads and attach another set of electrodes.

- **Water.** Move the victim out of freestanding fresh- or saltwater before attaching the AED. Water or sweat on the victim's chest may also conduct energy from one electrode pad to the other, reducing the potential for a successful shock. If the victim's chest is wet, sweaty, or dirty, quickly clean and dry it before attaching the AED.

- **Medication patches.** Remove medication patches and wipe the skin area clean before attaching the AED electrode pads. Medication patches left in place may block the shock and can cause small burns to the skin.

- **Implanted medical devices.** Pacemakers and implantable cardioverter defibrillators (ICDs) can interfere with the use of an AED. Place electrode pads at least 1 inch (2.5 centimeters) away from an implanted device. Look for a lump beneath the skin of the upper chest or abdomen. If the victim is receiving internal shocks from the ICD (which looks similar to muscles contracting from external shocks from an AED), allow 30 to 60 seconds for the ICD to complete its cycle before attaching the AED. Rescuers touching the victim will not be harmed if the implanted device discharges.[46]

- **Oxygen.** Do not use oxygen when delivering shocks with an AED. There have been reports of victims and their bedding being set on fire during defibrillation.[47] The oxygen concentration necessary for producing ignition will typically extend less than a foot (30 centimeters) in any direction and will quickly disperse when removed. Therefore, you should remove the mask and place it several feet from the victim or shut off the oxygen flow when delivering shocks. Leaving a device that continues to discharge oxygen near the victim's head before defibrillation is dangerous.[48]

Metal surfaces pose no shock hazard to either you or the victim. Cell phones do not interfere with the AED. Always follow the manufacturer's recommended safety precautions.

Procedures for AED Use

Expose the victim's chest, turn on the AED, and immediately attach it to the victim. Whenever possible, position it next to the rescuer who will be operating it. If feasible, continue CPR while the pads are being applied. Listen carefully and follow the machine's instructions. See figure 4.22. For an unwitnessed cardiac arrest, local protocol may instruct EMS providers to provide a couple minutes of CPR to oxygenate the heart and brain before attempting defibrillation.[43]

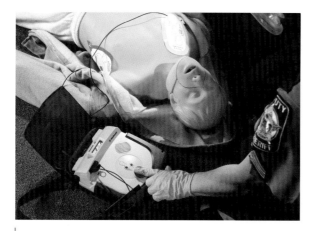

Figure 4.22 Using an AED for an adult victim.

AEDs may be used not only for adults but also for children older than 1 year who have no signs of life. See the pediatric defibrillator in figure 4.23. Some AED pads may require that the rescuer place one pad on the child's chest and one on the back. Always look at the pictures on the pads and place them as shown. You may need to use different cables or insert a key or turn a switch to deliver a lower amount of electricity for a child.[44,45] If a child-specific AED is not available, use a standard AED.

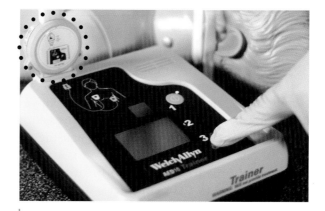

Figure 4.23 AED with Pediatric energy reducer.
Courtesy of Welch Allyn®, Inc.

Attaching and Operating an AED

AEDs are very easy to use. Research has shown that people can use AEDs adequately and safely without **any** instruction.[49-51] However, getting as little as 15 minutes of training will significantly improve your ability to operate an AED.[52, 53] Health care providers, first responders, and professional rescuers should practice CPR and AED as a team to make sure their actions are well timed and effective. ASHI recommends that a review of skills and practice drills for infrequent users occur about every 6 months. An AED program should be part of an overall system of quality assurance that includes medical oversight, training, data collection, and evaluation.

Many different brands of AEDs exist, but the same basic steps apply to all of them. If the victim is unresponsive and not breathing adequately, follow these steps.

1. Turn on the AED. Turning on the AED activates the voice prompts. Bare the victim's chest.

2. Follow the voice and visual prompts. Remove the disposable electrode pads from the packaging. Make sure to choose the correct pads (adult or child). **Do not use the child pads or system for an adult.** Look at the graphic images on each

electrode as a guide for proper pad placement. Remove the self-adhesive backing and attach the electrodes to the victim's bare chest. Make sure the electrodes attach firmly to the skin. Do not apply the pads over a female's breast, because it might decrease effectiveness.[54] Most AEDs will automatically begin to analyze a victim's heart rhythm when the electrodes are fully attached. Some will prompt you to push a button to analyze. Ensure that nobody touches the victim while the AED is analyzing the heart rhythm.

3. Follow procedures for shock or no shock. If a shock is indicated, check to make sure no one is touching the victim. Loudly say, "Clear!" or something similar. Push the shock button and immediately resume chest compressions. If no shock is indicated, immediately resume chest compressions. Perform 5 cycles of 30 compressions and 2 breaths and then very briefly reassess the rhythm. Continue as directed by the AED.

Research shows that errors by AED operators do occur. These include interference in AED operation by unnecessary movement (CPR during rhythm analysis), inappropriately turning the AED off, pads falling off or being disconnected, shockable rhythm not shocked, inappropriate shock delivered, and interference from movement other than CPR.[55,56] Very few rhythms are mismanaged by AEDs. AED operators must listen carefully and follow the AED's prompts.

Troubleshooting an AED

If an AED detects a problem during use, a voice or visual prompt, screen message, or lit icon will be displayed. Stay calm and do what the AED tells you to do. Here are some examples:

- If a message indicating motion occurs, make sure the cables are not being moved around.
- If a message regarding the battery is displayed, the battery power is probably low. The AED will prompt you to change the battery.

Maintenance and Quality Assurance

AEDs perform regular self-tests to make sure they are ready for use. If an AED fails a self-test, it will alert you with an audible or visual prompt. Contact authorized service personnel immediately. Inspect AEDs monthly. If the AED has a visual status indicator, check it to make sure it shows the device is operational. Examine the expiration dates on pad packages and spare batteries and inspect the AED for obvious damage. Make sure the battery and a replacement battery (or batteries) are fully operational and ready to use.

Store AEDs with the necessary equipment to respond to a cardiac arrest. The equipment should include the following, at a minimum:

- Personal protective equipment (CPR shield or mask and disposable gloves)
- Utility scissors (to cut clothing and expose chest)
- A disposable razor (to shave a hairy chest)
- Disposable towels (to dry the chest)
- A plastic biohazard bag (to dispose of used supplies)

CAUTION!

Never push the Analyze button when moving a victim on a stretcher or in an ambulance with an AED attached. It may simulate ventricular fibrillation. Stop movement and then analyze.

Rescue Breathing With Bag-Mask Device for Adults and Children

One Rescuer

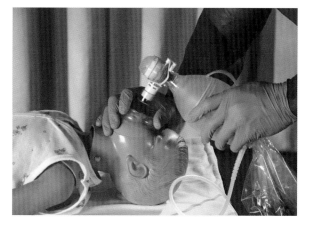

A = Airway

1. Position yourself above the victim's head. Place a mask on the face.
2. Place the thumb and first finger of one hand around the valve in a C position to press the mask against the face.
3. Use your remaining 3 fingers in an E position to lift up on the jaw.
4. Tilt the head back to open the airway. If the victim is injured, use a jaw thrust.

B = Breathing

1. Squeeze the bag with your free hand to ventilate. Give each breath in 1 second. Make the chest visibly rise.

   Adult rescue breathing: 1 breath every 5 to 6 seconds

   Child rescue breathing: 1 breath every 3 to 5 seconds
2. Watch for the chest to rise with each ventilation.

Two or More Rescuers

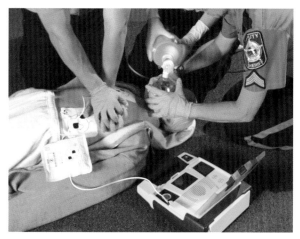

A = Airway (Rescuer 1)

1. Position yourself above the victim's head. Place a mask on the face.
2. Place the thumb and first finger of **each** hand around the valve in a C position. Press the mask against the face.
3. Use the remaining fingers on **each** hand in an E position to lift up on the jaw.
4. Tilt the head back to open the airway. If the victim is injured, use a jaw thrust.
5. Watch for the chest to rise with each ventilation.

B = Breathing (Rescuer 2)

1. Squeeze the bag to ventilate. Give each breath in 1 second. Make the chest visibly rise.

   Adult rescue breathing: 1 breath every 5 to 6 seconds

   Child rescue breathing: 1 breath every 3 to 5 seconds
2. Watch for the chest to rise with each ventilation.

Advanced Airways in Place

Give 1 breath every 6 to 8 seconds.

Adult CPR and AED for Single or Multiple Rescuers

Steps and procedures should occur simultaneously with two or more rescuers.

Emergency Action Steps

1. **Assess scene.** If the scene is not safe or at any time becomes unsafe, **get out!**
2. **Assess victim.** Not moving? No response?
3. **Alert.** Shout for help. No help? Alert EMS or activate emergency action plan, and get AED and oxygen.
4. **Attend to the ABCDs.**

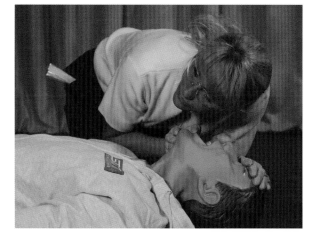

A = Airway: Open Airway

- Tilt head and lift chin.
- If the victim is injured, use a jaw thrust.

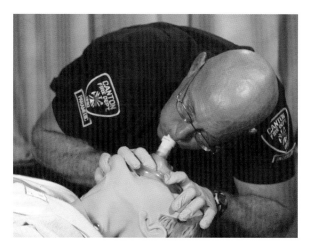

B = Breathing: Check Breathing

- Look, listen, and feel for 5, but no more than 10, seconds.
- If the victim is not breathing, give 2 breaths that make the chest visibly rise.

C = Circulation: Check Pulse

Check the carotid pulse for 5, but no more than 10, seconds.

- If there is a definite pulse, do the following:
  - Perform rescue breathing.
  - Give 1 breath every 5 to 6 seconds.

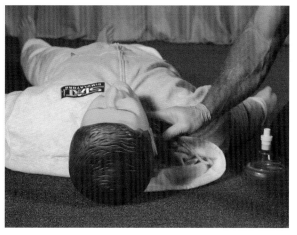

(continued)

Adult CPR and AED for Single or Multiple Rescuers

- **If there is no pulse or you are uncertain, immediately start chest compressions.**
  - If one rescuer, give 30 chest compressions, then 2 rescue breaths (30:2).
    - Give 30 compressions in middle of chest between the nipples.
    - Push hard and fast (100 times per minute). Allow the chest to recoil completely. Minimize interruptions.
    - Continue 30:2 until an AED or EMS or advanced providers arrive or the victim shows signs of life.

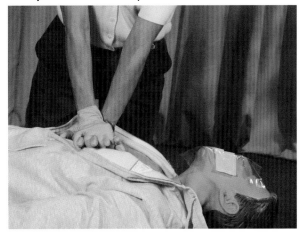

  - If two or more rescuers, give 30 chest compressions, then 2 rescue breaths (30:2).
    - Rescuer 1: Give 30 chest compressions.
    - Rescuer 2: Give 2 rescue breaths. Make the chest visibly rise.
    - Quickly change positions every 5 cycles (2 minutes).

Advanced Airways in Place

- Give 1 breath every 6 to 8 seconds.
- Give compressions 100 times a minute. Don't pause for breaths.

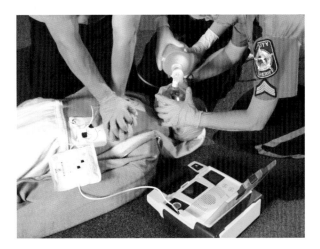

D = Defibrillation

- Expose the chest and turn on the AED. Select and attach the **adult** pads. Follow the voice prompts:
  - **Shock** advised: **Clear** and give 1 shock. Immediately resume chest compressions.
  - **No shock** advised: Immediately resume chest compressions.
- Continue 30 compressions, 2 breaths × 5 cycles. Check the rhythm, continue CPR and AED until advanced providers take over.

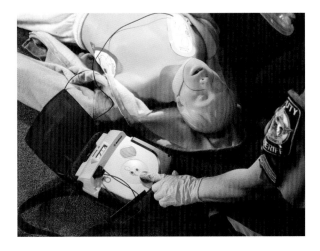

Child CPR and AED for Single or Multiple Rescuers

Steps and procedures should occur simultaneously with two or more rescuers.

Emergency Action Steps

1. **Assess scene.** If the scene is not safe or at any time becomes unsafe, **get out!**
2. **Assess victim.** Not moving? No response?
3. **Alert.** Shout for help. Send help to alert EMS or activate emergency action plan and get an AED and oxygen.
4. **Attend to the ABCDs.**

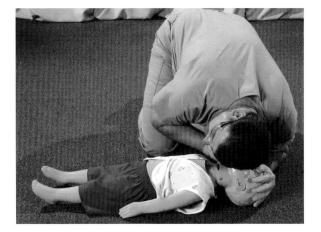

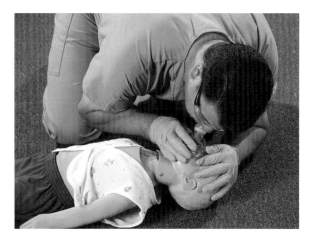

A = Airway: Open Airway

- Tilt head and lift chin.
- If the victim is injured, use a jaw thrust.

B = Breathing: Check Breathing

- Look, listen, and feel for 5, but no more than 10, seconds.
- If the victim is not breathing, give 2 breaths that make the chest visibly rise.

C = Circulation: Check Pulse

- Check pulse for 5, but no more than 10, seconds.
- If there is a **definite pulse,** perform rescue breathing. Give 1 breath every 3 to 5 seconds.

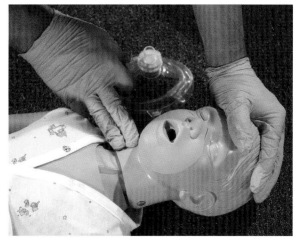

(continued)

Child CPR and AED for Single or Multiple Rescuers

- If there is **no pulse, the pulse is less than 60 BPM with poor color, or you are uncertain,** immediately start chest compressions and use the following procedures:
  - If one rescuer, give 30 chest compressions, then 2 rescue breaths (30:2).
    - Give 30 chest compressions in middle of chest between the nipples.
    - Push hard and fast (100 times per minute). Allow the chest to recoil completely.
    - Minimize interruptions.
    - Continue 30 compressions, 2 breaths × 5 cycles. Alert EMS; get an AED and oxygen if alone.
  - If two or more rescuers, give 15 chest compressions, then 2 rescue breaths (15:2).
    - Rescuer 1: Give 15 chest compressions.
    - Rescuer 2: Give 2 rescue breaths. Make the chest visibly rise.
    - Quickly change positions every 5 cycles (2 minutes).

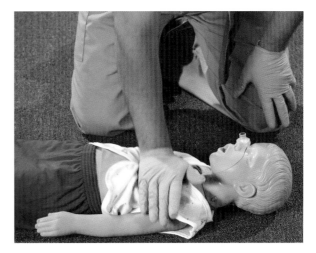

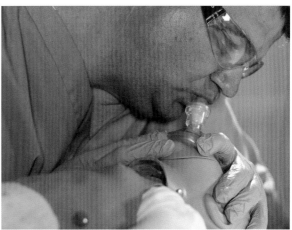

Advanced Airways in Place

- Give 1 breath every 6 to 8 seconds.
- Give compressions 100 times a minute. Don't pause for breaths.

D = Defibrillation

- Expose the victim's chest and turn on the AED. Select and attach the child pads and system (if not available, use the adult pads or system). Follow the voice prompts:
  - **Shock** advised: **Clear** and give 1 shock. Immediately resume chest compressions.
  - **No shock** advised: Immediately resume chest compressions.
- Continue CPR for 5 cycles (2 minutes). Check rhythm.

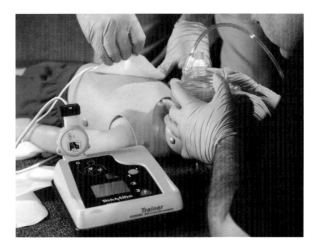

Rescue Breathing With Bag-Mask Device for Infants

One Rescuer

A = Airway

- Position yourself above the victim's head.
- Place the mask over the nose and mouth. Do not cover the eyes or chin.
- Use the thumb and first finger of one hand around the valve in a C position to press the mask against the face.
- Use your remaining 3 fingers in an E position to lift up on the jaw.
- Tilt the head back to open the airway. If the victim is injured, use a jaw thrust.

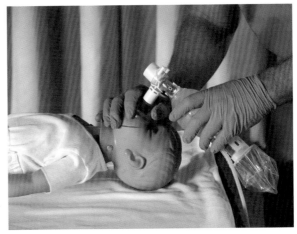

B = Breathing

- Squeeze the bag with your free hand to ventilate.
- Give each breath in 1 second. Make the chest visibly rise.
- Give 1 breath every 3 to 5 seconds (12 to 20 per minute).

Two or More Rescuers

A = Airway (Rescuer 1)

- Position yourself above the victim's head.
- Place the mask over the nose and mouth. Do not cover the eyes or chin.
- Use the thumb and first finger of one hand around the valve in a C position to press the mask against the face.
- Use your remaining 3 fingers in an E position to lift up on the jaw.
- Tilt the head back to open the airway. If the victim is injured, use a jaw thrust.
- Watch for the chest to rise with each ventilation.

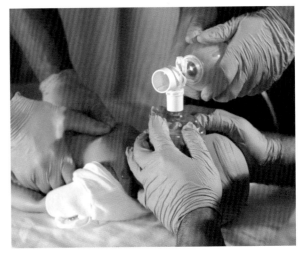

B = Breathing (Rescuer 2)

- Squeeze the bag to ventilate.
- Give each breath in 1 second. Make the chest visibly rise.
- Give 1 breath every 3 to 5 seconds (12 to 20 per minute).
- Check the pulse about every 2 minutes.

Advanced Airways in Place

- Give 1 breath every 6 to 8 seconds (8 to 10 breaths per minute).
- Check the pulse about every 2 minutes.

Infant CPR for Single or Multiple Rescuers

Steps and procedures should occur simultaneously with two or more rescuers.

Emergency Action Steps

1. **Assess scene.** If the scene is not safe or at any time becomes unsafe, **get out!**
2. **Assess victim.** Not moving? No response?
3. **Alert.** Shout for help. Send help to alert EMS or emergency action plan and get oxygen.
4. **Attend to the ABCs.**

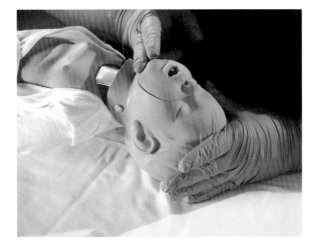

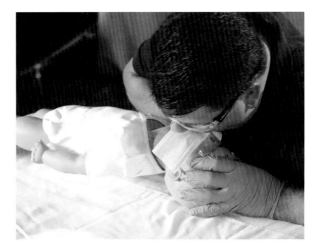

A = Airway: Open Airway

- Tilt head and lift chin.
- If the victim is injured, use a jaw thrust.

B = Breathing: Check Breathing

- Look, listen, and feel for 5, but no more than 10, seconds.
- If the victim is not breathing, give 2 breaths that make the chest visibly rise.

C = Circulation: Check Pulse

- Check the brachial pulse for 5, but no more than 10, seconds.
- If there is a **definite pulse,** perform rescue breathing. Give 1 breath every 3 to 5 seconds.

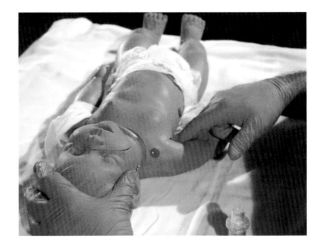

- If there is **no pulse, the pulse is less than 60 BPM with poor color, or you are uncertain,** immediately start chest compressions and use the following procedures:

  - If one rescuer, give 30 chest compressions, then 2 rescue breaths (30:2).

    - Give 30 chest compressions using 2 fingertips just below the nipple line.
    - Push hard and fast (100 times per minute).
    - Allow the chest to recoil completely. Minimize interruptions.
    - Continue 30 compressions, 2 breaths × 5 cycles. Alert EMS if alone.

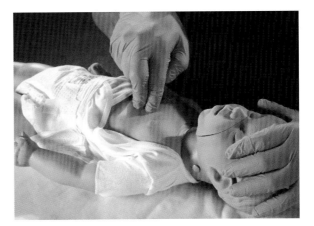

  - If two or more rescuers, give 15 chest compressions, then 2 rescue breaths (15:2).

    - Rescuer 1: Give 15 chest compressions using 2 thumbs with the fingers encircling the chest.
    - Rescuer 2: Give 2 rescue breaths. Make the chest visibly rise.
    - Quickly change positions every 5 cycles (2 minutes).

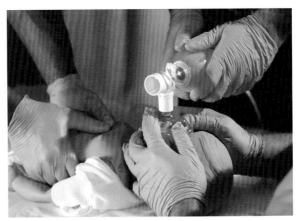

Advanced Airways in Place

- Give 1 breath every 6 to 8 seconds.
- Compressions 100 times a minute. Don't pause for breaths.

Summary of Basic Life Support Procedures

Table 4.1 summarizes the BLS procedures for adults, children, and infants.

Table 4.1   Basic Life Support Procedures for Adults, Children, and Infants

	Adult (about onset of puberty)	Child (about 1 year to onset of puberty)	Infant (less than about 1 year)
Assess			
Scene	If the scene is not safe or at any time becomes unsafe, **get out!**	If the scene is not safe or at any time becomes unsafe, **get out!**	If the scene is not safe or at any time becomes unsafe, **get out!**
Victim	Check for response. If victim is unresponsive or not moving, continue to alert step.	Check for response. If victim is unresponsive or not moving, continue to alert step.	Check for response. If victim is unresponsive or not moving, continue to alert step.
Alert: EMS or the emergency action plan.	**Alert** as soon as victim is found.	Give about 5 cycles of CPR, then **alert.**	Give about 5 cycles of CPR, then **alert.**
Attend to the ABCDs			
Airway: Open airway.	Tilt head, lift chin. If injury, do a jaw thrust.	Tilt head, lift chin. If injury, do a jaw thrust.	Tilt head, lift chin. If injury, do a jaw thrust.
Breathing: Look, listen, and feel for at least 5, but no more than 10, seconds.	**Initial:** 2 rescue breaths (ventilation without compression). Give each breath in 1 second. Make chest visibly rise. **Rescue breathing only:** About 1 breath every 5 to 6 seconds. **Advanced airway in place:** 1 breath every 6 to 8 seconds (8 to 10 breaths per minute).	**Initial:** 2 rescue breaths (ventilation without compression). Give each breath in 1 second. Make chest visibly rise. **Rescue breathing only:** About 1 breath every 3 to 5 seconds. **Advanced airway in place:** 1 breath every 6 to 8 seconds (8 to 10 breaths per minute).	**Initial:** 2 rescue breaths (ventilation without compression). Give each breath in 1 second. Make chest visibly rise. **Rescue breathing only:** About 1 breath every 3 to 5 seconds. **Advanced airway in place:** 1 breath every 6 to 8 seconds (8 to 10 breaths per minute).
Circulation: Check pulse for 5, but no more than 10, seconds.	Carotid (neck).	Carotid (neck) or femoral (groin).	Brachial (inside upper arm).
Compressions			
Position	In center of chest, between nipples, use 2 hands.	In center of chest, between nipples, use 1 or 2 hands.	**One rescuer:** Use 2 fingers, just below nipple line. **Two or more rescuers:** Use 2 thumbs with fingers encircling chest.
Method	Hard, fast, complete recoil, minimize interruption.	Hard, fast, complete recoil, minimize interruption.	Hard, fast, complete recoil, minimize interruption.

Depth	1.5 to 2 inches (4 to 5 centimeters).	About one-third to one-half depth of chest.	About one-third to one-half depth of chest.
Speed	About 100 times a minute.	About 100 times a minute.	About 100 times a minute.
Ratio	30:2	**One rescuer: 30:2.** **Two or more rescuers: 15:2.**	**One rescuer: 30:2.** **Two or more rescuers: 15:2.**
Defibrillation (AED)			
Operation	Expose chest, turn on AED. Select and attach **adult** pads. Follow voice prompts.	Expose chest, turn on AED. Select and attach **child** pads or system. Follow voice prompts.	No recommendations.
Type	Standard AED. Do **not** use child system.	Use **child** pads and system. If not available, use a standard AED.	No recommendations.

Choking (Foreign-Body Airway Obstruction)

Coughing is the body's way of trying to remove a foreign object (such as food) from the throat. If coughing does not clear the object, then choking occurs. Choking is an emergency that will result in unconsciousness and brain death within minutes if left untreated.

Children are particularly at risk for choking because of the small size of their air passages, inexperience with chewing, and a natural tendency to put objects in their mouths. In children ages 5 to 14 years, the majority of choking episodes are associated with food, especially candy. See figure 4.24. For children ages 1 to 4 years, coins are involved in 18% of all choking-related emergencies.[57] Peanuts and other nuts also are common causes of choking.[58] Children under 3 years of age should never be fed nuts or other hard, crunchy foods.[59]

Adults commonly choke on large pieces of food, often while drinking alcohol. Elderly persons frequently choke on semisolid foods.[60] When the air passages are blocked, the victim

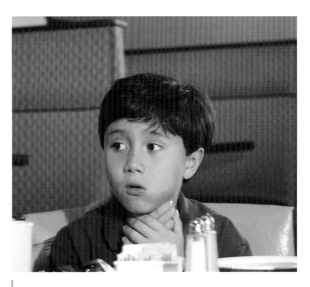

Figure 4.24   Child choking.

cannot breathe. Rapid first aid for choking can save a life. Table 4.2 shows the signs and symptoms and treatment guidelines for dealing with choking adults, children, and infants.

Table 4.2 Signs and Symptoms and Treatment for Choking

Adults and children older than 1 year

| Air exchange is good (mild blockage) | |
Signs and symptoms	Treatment guidelines
• Conscious or responsive • Can breathe in and out and can speak • Strong coughing or gagging as food or liquid "goes down the wrong pipe" • May hear high-pitched squeaking or whistling noise (wheezing) between strong coughs	• Encourage the victim to cough. • Stay with the victim. • Watch the victim closely. • Be ready to take action if symptoms worsen. • If blockage continues, alert EMS. *Note:* An incomplete obstruction of the airway may have less severe symptoms and be confused with other causes of upper-airway obstruction such as reactive airway disease (asthma) or croup. If the victim is coughing forcefully, help him or her into a comfortable position. Call EMS or activate emergency action plan.

| Air exchange is poor or nonexistent (severe blockage) | | |
	Signs and symptoms	Treatment guidelines
Responsive	• Clutching throat • Cannot cough or make any sound • Blue lips, nails, skin	• Quickly ask, "Are you choking?" If the victim nods yes or is unable to speak, cough, or cry, **act quickly!** • Stand behind an adult or kneel behind a child. • Make a fist. Place the thumb side against the victim's abdomen, just above the navel. • Give quick inward and upward thrusts until the object is expelled or the victim becomes unresponsive. (See Skill Guide 6.)
Late stages of pregnancy or obese		• Perform chest thrusts. Stand behind the victim. Place your arms under the victim's armpits, encircling the chest. Place the thumb side of your fist on the middle of the sternum. • Grasp your fist with your other hand and thrust backward. Continue until the object is expelled or the victim becomes unresponsive.
Self		• Give yourself abdominal thrusts until the object is expelled. • If that does not work, quickly press your abdomen over any firm surface (back of a chair, side of a table).
Unresponsive		• Carefully get the adult to the ground, immediately alert EMS, or activate emergency action plan. If you are alone with a child, give about 5 cycles (2 minutes) of CPR, then alert EMS. • Open the airway. Remove the object if you see it. Begin CPR. • Each time you open the airway for rescue breaths, look for an object in the victim's throat. If you see it, remove it. • Continue CPR until the AED or EMS arrives or the victim shows signs of life.

Caution!

Abdominal thrusts have been associated with severe and fatal complications. Complications may occur even when abdominal thrusts are performed correctly. **Do not** perform the Heimlich maneuver on an adult or child unless it is necessary. A victim who had an airway obstruction that was removed by abdominal or chest thrusts should be evaluated by a physician to ensure no internal injuries resulted from the event.

Infants

	Air exchange is good (mild blockage)	
	Signs and symptoms	Treatment guidelines
Responsive	• Can breathe in and out • Crying, gagging • Strong coughing • May hear high-pitched whistling or squeaking noise (wheezing) between strong coughs	• Stay with the victim. • Watch the victim closely. • Be ready to take action if the symptoms worsen. • If the blockage continues, alert EMS.
	Air exchange is poor or nonexistent (severe blockage)	
	Signs and symptoms	Treatment guidelines
Responsive	• Cannot cough or make any sound • Blue lips, nails, skin • Passing out	• Keep the infant's head lower than the chest. • Give 5 back slaps between the shoulder blades with enough force to expel the object. • Turn the infant faceup onto your lap or thigh. • Give 5 downward chest thrusts just below the nipple line with enough force to expel the object. • Repeat until the object is expelled or the infant becomes unresponsive.
Unresponsive		• Place the infant on a firm, flat surface. Open the airway. • Remove the object if you see it. Begin CPR. • Each time you open the airway for rescue breaths, look for an object in the infant's throat. If you see it, carefully remove it. • Do not blindly sweep your finger through an infant or child's throat. Blind finger sweeps can cause injury and push the object deeper into the airway.[61, 62] • Continue CPR for about 2 minutes (5 cycles). Alert EMS or activate emergency action plan.

Caution!
The Heimlich maneuver is not recommended for infants because it may damage internal organs. An infant who had an airway obstruction that was removed by back slaps or chest thrusts should be evaluated by EMS and seen by a physician to ensure no internal injuries resulted from the event.

Adult or Child Choking: Severe Blockage

Emergency Action Steps
Assess, alert, and attend to the ABCs.

Responsive

- Victim is clutching throat and cannot cough or make any sound.
- Quickly ask, "Are you choking?"
- If the victim nods yes or is unable to speak, cough, or cry, act quickly.
- Stand behind an adult or kneel behind a child.
- Make a fist. Place the thumb side against the victim's abdomen, just above the navel.
- Give quick inward and upward thrusts until the object is expelled or the victim becomes unresponsive.

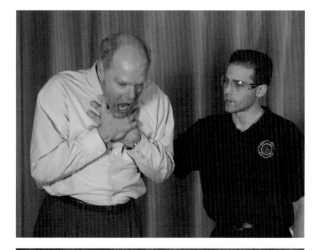

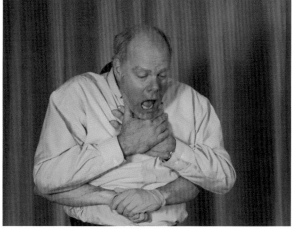

Unresponsive

- Carefully get the victim to the ground and immediately activate EMS or the emergency action plan. If you are alone with a child, give about 5 cycles (2 minutes) of CPR, then alert EMS.
- Open the airway. Remove the object if you see it.
- Begin CPR.
- Each time you open the airway for rescue breaths, look for an object in the victim's throat. If you see it, remove it.
- Continue CPR until an AED or EMS arrives or the victim shows signs of life.

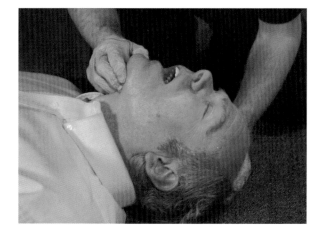

Infant Choking: Severe Blockage

Emergency Action Steps
Assess, alert, and attend to the ABCs.

Responsive

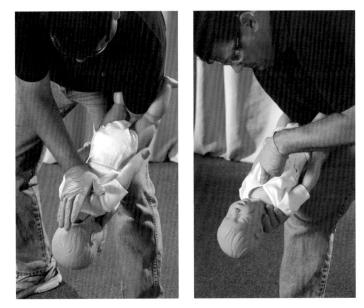

- Infant cannot cough, cry, or make any sound.
- Rest the infant facedown on your forearm. Place your forearm on your lap or thigh.
- Keep the infant's head lower than the chest. Support the head and the jaw with your hand.
- Give 5 back blows or slaps between the shoulder blades with enough force to expel the object.
- Support the head and the neck and turn the infant over (faceup) onto your lap or thigh.
- Give 5 downward chest thrusts just below the nipple line with enough force to expel the object.
- Repeat until the object is expelled or the infant becomes unresponsive.

Unresponsive

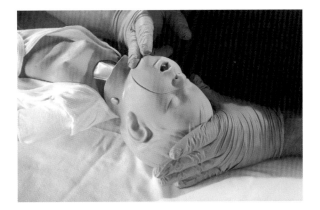

- Place the infant on a firm, flat surface.
- Open the airway. Remove the object if you see it.
- Begin CPR.
- Each time you open the airway for rescue breaths, look for an object in the infant's throat. If you see it, remove it.
- Do not blindly sweep your finger through an infant or child's throat.
- Continue CPR for about 2 minutes (5 cycles). Alert EMS or activate your emergency action plan.

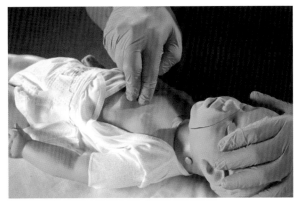

Psychological and Legal Aspects of Providing Basic Life Support

People trained in CPR are often unwilling to perform it. They give a variety of reasons, including fear of disease, fear of hurting the victim, fear of performing the skills incorrectly, and fear of liability.[63, 64] The following are some of the psychological and legal aspects of providing basic life support.

Psychological Aspects

Fear of catching a disease from performing CPR is mostly unfounded. The risk of contracting a disease while giving CPR is extremely low, and observing universal precautions for victims of all ages will make it lower. Fears associated with CPR skill performance can be reduced through regular participation in training that focuses on simple, practical skills and confidence building. Still, when resuscitation is attempted, doctors, nurses, EMS providers, and bystanders can have a wide range of negative reactions and emotional stress.[65-68] Failed resuscitation attempts often leave laypersons and professionals (especially those who perform resuscitation infrequently) with feelings of guilt and failure when CPR was not done correctly.[69] This distress is normal and usually temporary.

Rib and breastbone fractures do occur frequently during chest compressions in adult CPR, but they are not major complications.[70] In infants and toddlers, CPR rarely causes such injuries.[71]

Although CPR should be done correctly, it is helpful to remember that a person in cardiac arrest is dead (without breathing or a pulse). It is difficult to make the person "worse." The root of the word *resuscitate* is from the Latin *revivere,* which means "to live again." Rescuers who perform good CPR in a good-faith attempt to give the victim a chance to live again should not hold themselves responsible when that attempt does not restore life fully—or at all. Mistakes in resuscitation may reduce the chances for successfully resuscitating victims, but the mistakes do not kill them. The majority of adult and child victims of cardiac arrest are not brought back to life.

Those who attempt CPR may also have traumatic stress reactions after they respond to a crisis. Traumatic stress reactions are a normal human response to a traumatic event and usually are temporary. Symptoms begin within minutes of the traumatic event and should disappear within hours or a couple days. Table 4.3 gives an overview of the traumatic stress reactions that rescuers may have after a rescue event and recommendations for addressing those reactions.

Legal and Ethical Aspects

A few key legal and ethical principles are involved when you provide basic life support, which are described in table 4.4.

Table 4.3 Traumatic Stress Reactions

	Signs and symptoms	Recommendations
During the incident	<ul><li>Anxiety or worry</li><li>Trembling or shaking</li><li>Sweating</li><li>Fast breathing</li><li>Pounding heartbeat, shock, anger</li><li>Excitement, intense fear</li><li>Nausea</li></ul>	<ul><li>Remain calm and act sensibly.</li><li>Accept your own limitations as a rescuer.</li></ul>
After the incident	<ul><li>Repeated thoughts or flashbacks of event</li><li>Worry about self or loved ones</li><li>Guilt for not having done more or better</li><li>Tense muscles, diarrhea or constipation, nausea or vomiting, headaches, fatigue</li><li>Avoiding reminders of incident</li><li>Easily startled</li><li>Lack of interest in usual activities</li><li>Sadness, feeling numb or detached</li><li>Sleep problems or nightmares</li><li>Problems concentrating</li><li>Hyperactive or depressed</li></ul>	<ul><li>Remind yourself that stress reactions are normal and will pass.</li><li>Get back into a normal routine as soon as possible.</li><li>Be kind to yourself. Allow yourself time to deal with memories of the incident.</li><li>Accept every person's right to his or her own feelings.</li><li>Keep what happened in a realistic perspective.</li><li>Exercise, eat, drink, and rest.</li><li>Have a connection to professional resources for continued care if necessary.</li></ul>

Table 4.4 Legal and Ethical Principles of Basic Life Support

Principle	Key points
Good Samaritan principle and laws	• Based on the Biblical story. Prevents a rescuer who has voluntarily helped a stranger in need from being sued for wrongdoing. • In most of North America you have no legal obligation to help a person in need.[a] Since governments encourage people to help others, they pass Good Samaritan laws (or apply the principle to common laws). • You are generally protected from liability as long as you are reasonably careful, act in good faith (not for reward), and do not provide care beyond your skill level. • If you decide to help an ill or injured person, you must not leave that person until someone with equal or more emergency training takes over (unless it becomes dangerous to stay).
Consent	• *Consent* means permission. A responsive adult must agree to receive care. • *Expressed consent* means the victim gives his or her permission to receive care. To get consent, first identify yourself. Then tell the victim your level of training and ask if it's OK to help. • *Implied consent* means that permission to perform care on an unresponsive victim is assumed. This is based on the idea that a reasonable person would give permission to receive lifesaving care if he or she were able. • **Children:** Consent must be gained from a parent or legal guardian. When life-threatening situations exist and a parent or legal guardian is not available, care should be given based on implied consent. • **Elderly:** If suffering from a disturbance in normal mental functioning, such as Alzheimer's disease, a victim may not understand your request for consent. Consent must be gained from a family member or legal guardian.
Duty to act	• *Duty to act* is a requirement to act toward others and the public with the watchfulness, attention, caution, and prudence that a reasonable person in the same circumstances would use. • If a person's actions do not meet this standard, then the acts may be considered negligent, and any damages resulting may be claimed in a lawsuit for negligence.[72] If you are a state-licensed health care provider, first responder, or other professional rescuer expected to give emergency medical care, including CPR, you almost certainly have a duty to act. However, BLS performed voluntarily on a stranger in need while you are off duty is generally considered a Good Samaritan act.

Starting and stopping CPR	Start CPR for all victims in cardiac arrest unless
	
	• signs of irreversible death are present, including the following:
	  - Rigor mortis (limbs of the corpse are stiff and impossible to move)
	  - Lividity (settling of blood in the lower portions of the body, causing a purplish red discoloration)
	  - Conditions incompatible with life (decomposition, decapitation, massive head injury)
	• providing CPR would put the rescuer in danger of injury,
	• victim has a valid DNR order (see section at end of table), or
	• there are many victims (for example, in a catastrophic natural disaster or terrorist attack).
	
	A victim who is not breathing after two attempts to open the airway is considered dead. This is because the time required to provide CPR and external chest compressions is not justified when there are many victims needing first aid.
	
	Do not stop CPR until any of the following conditions occur:
	
	• A health care provider or other professional rescuer with equal or more training takes over or the victim shows signs of life.
	• You are exhausted.
	• The scene becomes too dangerous to continue.
	• The doctor in charge of the victim decides to order the resuscitation effort stopped (follow local protocol, standard operating procedures, or medical direction).
	
	Note: Except when death is obvious, irreversible brain damage or brain death cannot be reliably assessed or predicted.[73] Rescuers should never make an impulsive decision about the present or future quality of life of a cardiac arrest victim because such decisions are often incorrect.

Advance directives and living wills	• These are documents authorized by state law and are usually witnessed or notarized. Also called a *durable power of attorney.* • The documents allow a person to appoint someone as his or her representative to make decisions on resuscitation and continued life support if the person has lost his or her decision-making capacity (for example, if he or she is in a coma). • Advance directives are statements about what victims want done or not done if they can't speak for themselves. • Laws about advance directives are different in each state. You should be aware of the laws in your state.
Do not resuscitate (DNR) or do not attempt resuscitation (DNAR) orders	• The DNR or DNAR order is a type of advance directive. This is a specific request not to have CPR performed. • In the United States, a doctor's order is required to withhold CPR. Therefore, unless the victim has a DNR order, EMS providers and hospital staff should attempt resuscitation. • Victims who are not likely to benefit from CPR and may have a DNR order include those with terminal conditions from which they are unlikely to recover. • Outside the hospital, health care providers, first responders, and other professional rescuers should begin CPR if there is a reasonable doubt about the validity of a DNAR order or advance directive, the victim may have changed his or her mind, or the victim's best interests may be in question.[74]

ª There are exceptions. Two U.S. states (Vermont and Minnesota) and one Canadian province (Quebec) have failure-to-act laws that require all citizens to assist a victim in need as long as they don't endanger their own lives.

Special Conditions

The following conditions may or may not require changes in standard CPR procedures. However, each condition requires some special consideration. See table 4.5 for specific considerations.

Table 4.5   Specific Considerations for Special Conditions

Condition	Changes or special considerations
Pregnancy	**Assess scene and victim: no change. A = airway: no change. B = breathing: no change. C = circulation: change.** Chest compressions may not be effective when a woman who is 6 months pregnant or more is lying flat on her back. This is because the baby puts pressure on the major vein that returns blood to the heart. If possible, prop up the victim slightly on her left side using a rolled blanket (or something similar) when performing chest compressions. This reduces the pressure and provides the most blood flow to the mother and baby. Perform chest compressions higher on the breastbone, slightly above the center. **D = defibrillation: no change.**
Hypothermia	**Assess scene and victim: change.** Get indoors or out of the wind. Prevent additional heat loss by removing wet clothes and insulating the victim from further exposure. If the victim's body is frozen solid, nose and mouth are blocked with ice, and chest compression is impossible, do not start CPR. **A = airway: no change. B = breathing: no change. C = circulation: no change. D = defibrillation: change.** If the victim does not respond to one shock, focus on continuing CPR and rewarming the victim to a range of 86 to 89.6 °F (30 to 32 °C) before repeating a defibrillation attempt.
Submersion or near drowning	**Assess scene and victim: change.** Caution! The scene may be unsafe (waves, currents, cold water, bad weather). Proper training and use of personal lifesaving equipment, such as rescue devices and personal flotation devices, are critical for a safe rescue. If a boat or other vessel is available, get the victim into it. If no boat is available, get the victim to the shore. Start BLS or CPR if indicated, as soon as it is safe to do so. **A = airway: no change. B = breathing: change.** Expect vomiting. When it occurs, turn the victim to the side and remove the vomit with a sweep of a gloved finger or cloth. If a head, neck, or back injury is suspected, use the HAINES method or roll the victim like a log. Minimize movement. Avoid twisting the head, neck, or back. Do not attempt to drain water from the lungs using abdominal thrusts or the Heimlich maneuver. It is unnecessary and potentially dangerous. **C = circulation: no change. D = defibrillation: change.** Move the victim out of freestanding water and dry the chest before attaching an AED.
Electric shock	**Assess scene and victim: change.** Consider any fallen or broken wire extremely dangerous. Do not touch (or allow your clothing to touch) a wire, victim, or vehicle that is possibly energized. Do not approach within 8 feet (2.4 meters) of it. Notify the local utility company and have trained personnel sent to the scene. Metal or cable guardrails, steel wire fences, and telephone lines may be energized by a fallen wire and may carry the current 1 mile (1.6 kilometers) or more from the point of contact. **Never** attempt to handle wires yourself unless you are properly trained and equipped.[75] Start BLS or CPR, if indicated, as soon as it is safe to do so. **A = airway: no change. B = breathing: no change. C = compressions: no change. D = defibrillation: no change.**

Lightning strike	Assess scene and victim: change. When multiple victims are struck by lightning at the same time, give the highest priority to those without signs of life. Start BLS or CPR, if indicated, as soon as it is safe to do so. Because many victims are young, they have a good chance for survival if CPR is given immediately. Remove smoldering clothing, shoes, and belts to prevent burns. A = airway: no change. B = breathing: no change. C = circulation: no change. D = defibrillation: no change.
Cardiac arrest and injury	Assess scene and victim: no change. A = airway: change. Clear mouth of blood, vomit, and other secretions. B = breathing: no change. C = circulation: no change. D = defibrillation: no change.
Family presence	Studies show that family members want to be present during a resuscitation attempt. Doing so may help them adjust to the death of their loved one and ease their own grieving. Other studies show that health care providers often disapprove of this practice, fearing psychological trauma to family members, legal concerns, and a fear of distracting the resuscitation team.[76] Despite this, there is evidence that when family is present there are fewer legal actions and less second-guessing about providers' competence. There apparently is no evidence that family presence is harmful.[77] Consequently, family presence during resuscitation is a reasonable and potentially desirable option.[78] An experienced health care provider, first responder, or other professional rescuer should be assigned to the family to answer questions, explain procedures, and offer comfort.[79] Both the providers and family should have a connection to professional counseling resources (clergy, crisis workers, social workers) for continued care if necessary.[80]

References

1. American Heart Association. Part 4: Adult basic life support. *Circulation* 2005; 112;IV-18-1V-34.

2. Madl C, Holzer M. Brain function after resuscitation from cardiac arrest. *Curr Opin Crit Care* 2004 June; 10(3):213-7.

3 Mejicano GC, Maki DG. Infections acquired during cardiopulmonary resuscitation: Estimating the risk and defining strategies for prevention. *Ann Intern Med.* 1998 November 15; 129(10):813-28.

4. U.S. Department of Health and Human Services, Centers for Disease Control and Prevention Center for Chronic Disease Prevention and Health Promotion. Preventing heart disease and stroke: Addressing the nation's leading killers. www.cdc.gov/nccdphp/aag/aag_cvd.htm. Accessed 2006 August.

5. Statistics Canada. Selected leading causes of death, by sex (1997). www40.statcan.ca/l01/cst01/health36.htm?sdi=causes%20death. Accessed 2006 September.

6. World Health Organization. The atlas of heart disease and stroke. www.who.int/cardiovascular_diseases/resources/atlas/en. Accessed 2006 August.

7. National Heart, Lung and Blood Institute (NHLBI). How can I prevent a heart attack? www.nhlbi.nih.gov/health/dci/Diseases/HeartAttack/HeartAttack_Prevention.html. Accessed 2006 August.

8. Merck & Co. The Merck manual of diagnoses and therapy. Section 16. Cardiovascular disorders, chapter 202: Coronary artery disease. www.merck.com/mrkshared/mmanual/section16/chapter202/202a.jsp. Accessed 2006 August.

9. National Institute of Neurological Disorders and Stroke, National Institutes of Health. August 7, 2006. NINDS stroke information page. www.ninds.nih.gov/disorders/stroke/stroke.htm. Accessed 2006 August.

10. Liferidge AT, Brice JH, Overby BA, Evenson KR. Ability of laypersons to use the Cincinnati Prehospital Stroke Scale. *Prehosp Emerg Care* 2004 October-December; 8(4):384-7.

11. American Heart Association. 2006. Learn to recognize a stroke. www.strokeassociation.org/presenter.jhtml?identifier=1020. Accessed 2006 August.

12. The Heart Rhythm Foundation. Sudden cardiac arrest key facts. www.heartrhythmfoundation.org/facts/scd.asp. Accessed 2006 September.

13. Medline Plus. Ventricular fibrillation. www.nlm.nih.gov/medlineplus/print/ency/article/007200.htm. Accessed 2005 19 October.

14. Heart Rhythm Society. Sudden cardiac death. www.hrspatients.org/patients/heart_disorders/cardiac_arrest/default.asp. Accessed 2006 August.

15. Newman MM. The chain of survival takes hold. *JEMS* 1989; 14(8):11-13.

16. Hau SR, et al. Factors impeding dispatcher-assisted telephone cardiopulmonary resuscitation. *Ann Emerg Med* 2003 December; 42(6):731-7.

17. Roppolo LP, et al. Council of Standards Pre-Arrival Instruction Committee, National Academies of Emergency Dispatch modified cardiopulmonary resuscitation (CPR) instruction protocols for emergency medical dispatchers: Rationale and recommendations. *Resuscitation* 2005 May; 65(2):203-10.

18. Valenzuela TD, Roe DJ, Nichol G, Clark LL, Spaite DW, Hardman RG. Outcomes of rapid defibrillation by security officers after cardiac arrest in casinos. *N Engl J Med* 2000 October 26; 343(17):1206-9.

19. Heart and Stroke Foundation of Canada. Chain of survival. http://ww1.heartandstroke.bc.ca/page.asp?PageID=388&LetterCode=67#Chain%20of%20survival. Accessed 2006 September.

20. Safe Kids Worldwide. Safety tips. www.safekids.org/tips/tips.html. Accessed 2006 August.

21. Thompson DC, Rivara FP. Pool fencing for preventing drowning in children. *Cochrane Database of Systematic Reviews* 1998; 1: CD001047. DOI: 10.1002/14651858.CD001047.

22. National Institute of Child Health and Human Development (NICHD). November 2005. SIDS: "Back to sleep" campaign. www.nichd.nih.gov/sids. Accessed 2006 August.

23. Hauck FR, Omojokun OO, Siadaty MS. Do pacifiers reduce the risk of sudden infant death syndrome? A meta-analysis. *Pediatrics* 2005 November; 116(5):e716-23.

24. Lopez-Herce J, et al. Long-term outcome of paediatric cardiorespiratory arrest in Spain. *Resuscitation* 2005 January; 64(1):79-85.

25. von Ungern-Sternberg BS, Erb TO, Frei FJ. Management of the upper airway in spontaneously breathing children: A challenge for the anaesthetist. *Anaesthetist* 2006 February; 55(2):164-70.

26. Hammer J, Reber A, Trachsel D, Frei FJ. Effect of jaw-thrust and continuous positive airway pressure on tidal breathing in deeply sedated infants. *J Pediatr* 2001 June; 138(6):826-30.

27 American Heart Association. 2006. *BLS for healthcare providers student manual.* Dallas, TX: American Heart Association.

28. Rathgeber J, et al. Influence of different types of recovery positions on perfusion indices of the forearm. *Resuscitation* 1996 July; 32(1):13-7.

29. Wenzel V, Idris AH, Banner MJ, Fuerst RS, Tucker KJ. The composition of gas given by mouth-to-mouth ventilation during CPR. *Chest* 1994 December; 106(6):1806-10.

30. Koksal N, Buyukbese MA, Guven A, Cetinkaya A, Hasanoglu HC. Organophosphate intoxication as a consequence of mouth-to-mouth breathing from an affected case. *Chest* 2002 August; 122(2):740-1.

31. U.S. Department of Labor Occupational Safety & Health Administration. Section 9-IX. Summary and explanation of the standard: Bloodborne pathogens (29CRF 1910.1030). www.osha.gov/pls/oshaweb/owadisp.show_document?p_table=PREAMBLES&p_id=811. Accessed 2006 August.

32. Le Conte P. June 21, 2006. Pneumonia, aspiration. www.emedicine.com/EMERG/topic464.htm. Accessed 2006 August.

33. Clark RK, Trethewy CE. Assessment of cricoid pressure application by emergency department staff. *Emerg Med Australas* 2005 August; 17(4):376-81.

34. Janda M, Vagts DA, Noldge-Schomburg GF. Cricoid pressure: Safety necessity or unnecessary risk? *Anaethesiol Reanim* 2004; 29(1):4-7.

35. Landsman, I. Cricoid pressure: Indications and complications *Pediatric Anaesthesia* 2004; 14:43-47.

36. Ewy GA. Cardiocerebral resuscitation: The new cardiopulmonary resuscitation. *Circulation* 2005 April 26; 111(16):2134-42.

37. Valenzuela TD et al. Interruptions of chest compressions during emergency medical systems resuscitation. *Circulation* 2005 August 30; 112(9):1259-65.

38. Kern KB, et al. Importance of continuous chest compressions during cardiopulmonary resuscitation: Improved outcome during a simulated single

lay-rescuer scenario. *Circulation* 2002 February 5; 105(5):645-9.

39. Hoke RS, Chamberlain D. Skeletal chest injuries secondary to cardiopulmonary resuscitation. *Resuscitation* 2004 December; 63(3):327-38.

40. Ashton A, McCluskey A, Gwinnutt CL, Keenan AM. Effect of rescuer fatigue on performance of continuous external chest compressions over 3 min. *Resuscitation* 2002 November; 55(2):151-5.

41. Hightower D, Thomas SH, Stone CK, Dunn K, March JA. Decay in quality of closed-chest compressions over time. *Ann Emerg Med* 1995 September; 26(3):300-3.

42. American Heart Association. Part 7.2: Management of cardiac arrest. *Circulation* 2005; 112: IV-18-IV-34.

43. Ewy GA. Cardiocerebral resuscitation: The new cardiopulmonary resuscitation. *Circulation* 2005 April 26; 111(16):2134-42.

44. Samson RA, et al. Use of automated external defibrillators for children: An update. An advisory statement from the pediatric advanced life support task force, International Liaison Committee on Resuscitation. *Circulation* 2003 July 1; 107(25):3250-5.

45. Atkins DL, Jorgenson DB. Attenuated pediatric electrode pads for automated external defibrillator use in children. *Resuscitation* 2005 July; 66(1):31-7.

46. Ganz, L. October 8, 2004. Implantable cardioverter/defibrillators. www.emedicine.com/med/topic3386.htm. Accessed 2006 August.

47. ECRI (formerly the Emergency Care Research Institute), Medical Devices Safety Reports. 2006. Fires from defibrillation during oxygen administration hazard. *Health Devices* July 1994; 23(7):307-8. www.mdsr.ecri.org/summary/detail.aspx?doc_id=8128. Accessed 2006 August.

48. Robertshaw H, McAnulty G. Ambient oxygen concentrations during simulated cardiopulmonary resuscitation. *Anaesthesia* 1998 July; 53(7):634-7.

49. Monsieurs KG, Vogels C, Bossaert LL, Meert P, Calle PA. A study comparing the usability of fully automatic versus semi-automatic defibrillation by untrained nursing students. *Resuscitation* 2005 January; 64(1): 41-7.

50. Sandroni C, et al. Automated external defibrillation by untrained deaf lay rescuers. *Resuscitation* 2004 October; 63(1): 43-8.

51. Wik L, Dorph E, Auestad B, Steen PA. Evaluation of a defibrillator-basic cardiopulmonary resuscitation programme for non medical personnel. *Resuscitation* 2003 February; 56(2): 167-72.

52. Callejas S, Barry A, Demertsidis E, Jorgenson D, Becker LB. Human factors impact successful lay person automated external defibrillator use during simulated cardiac arrest. *Crit Care Med* 2004 September; 32(9 Suppl):S406-13.

53. Beckers S, et al. Minimal instructions improve the performance of laypersons in the use of semiautomatic and automatic external defibrillators. *Crit Care* 2005 April; 9(2):R110-6.

54. Pagan-Carlo LA, Spencer KT, Robertson CE, Dengler A, Birkett C, Kerber RE. Transthoracic defibrillation: Importance of avoiding electrode placement directly on the female breast. *J Am Coll Cardiol* 1996; 27:449-452.

55. Macdonald RD, Swanson JM, Mottley JL, Weinstein C. Performance and error analysis of automated external defibrillator use in the out-of-hospital setting. *Ann Emerg Med* 2001 September; 38(3):262-7.

56. Ko PC, Lin CH, Lu TC, Ma MH, Chen WJ, Lin FY. Machine and operator performance analysis of automated external defibrillator utilization. *J Formos Med Assoc* 2005 July; 104(7):476-81.

57. U.S. Department of Health and Human Services, Centers for Disease Control and Prevention. Nonfatal choking-related episodes for children 0 to 14 years of age—United States, 2001. *Morbidity and Mortality Weekly Reports (MMWR)* 2002.

58. Chiu CY, Wong KS, Lai SH, Hsia SH, Wu CT. Factors predicting early diagnosis of foreign body aspiration in children. *Pediatr Emerg Care* 2005 March; 21(3):161-4.

59. Morley RE, et al. Foreign body aspiration in infants and toddlers: Recent trends in British Columbia. *J Otolaryngol* 2004 Feb; 33(1):37-41.

60. Berzlanovich AM. Foreign body asphyxia: A preventable cause of death in the elderly. *Am J Prev Med* 2005 January; 28(1):65-9.

61. Kabbani M, Goodwin SR. Traumatic epiglottis following blind finger sweep to remove a pharyngeal foreign body. *Clin Pediatr* 1995; 34:495-497.

62. Hartrey R, Bingham RM. Pharyngeal trauma as a result of blind finger sweeps in the choking child. *J Accid Emerg Med* 1995; 12:52-54.

63. 2005 International Liaison Committee on Resuscitation, American Heart Association, European

Resuscitation Council. Attitude toward performing CPR. 2005 International Consensus Conference on Cardiopulmonary Resuscitation and Emergency Cardiovascular Care Science with Treatment Recommendations. Dallas, TX, January 23-30, 2005. *Circulation* 2005; 112:III-100-III-108 and *Resuscitation* 2005 December; 67(1): S1-S190.

64. Shenefelt, R. Emotional aspects of basic life support. Presentation of Scientific Program of the New Zealand Resuscitation Council Conference, Wellington, NZ. November 1999.

65. Morgan R, Westmoreland C. Survey of junior hospital doctors' attitudes to cardiopulmonary resuscitation. *Postgrad Med J* 2002 July; 78(921):413-5.

66. Gamble M. A debriefing approach to dealing with the stress of CPR attempts. *Prof Nurse* 2001 November; 17(3):157-60.

67. Axelsson A, et al. Factors surrounding cardiopulmonary resuscitation influencing bystanders' psychological reactions. *Resuscitation* 1998 April; 37(1):13-20.

68. Swanson RW. Psychological issues in CPR. *Ann Emerg Med* 1993 February; 22(2 Pt 2):350-3.

69. Newman M. CPR comes full circle. *J Emerg Med Serv* 1990; 15(4):48-55.

70. Lederer W, Mair D, Rabl W, Baubin M. Frequency of rib and sternum fractures associated with out-of-hospital cardiopulmonary resuscitation is underestimated by conventional chest X-ray. *Resuscitation* 2004 February; 60(2):157-62.

71. Hoke RS, Chamberlain D. Skeletal chest injuries secondary to cardiopulmonary resuscitation. *Resuscitation* 2004 December; 63(3):327-38.

72. Law.com dictionary. http://dictionary.law.com/[28-Dec-05]

73. American Heart Association. Guidelines for cardiopulmonary resuscitation (CPR) and emergency cardiovascular care (ECC). Part 2: Ethical issues. *Circulation* 2005; 112.

74. American Heart Association. Part 2. Ethical Issues. Advance directives in the out-of-hospital setting. *Circulation* 2005; 112:IV-6-IV-11.

75. Bangor Hydro Electric Company. First responder safety. www.bhe.com/safety/responder.cfm. Accessed 2006 August.

76. McClenathan BM, Torrington KG, Uyehara CF. Family member presence during cardiopulmonary resuscitation: A survey of US and international critical care professionals. *Chest* 2002 December; 122(6):2204-11.

77. Nibert L, Ondrejka D. Family presence during pediatric resuscitation: An integrative review for evidence-based practice. *J Pediatr Nurs* 2005 April; 20(2):145-7.

78. Henderson DP, Knapp JF. Report of the National Consensus Conference on Family Presence During Pediatric Cardiopulmonary Resuscitation and Procedures. *Pediatr Emerg Care* 2005 November; 21(11):787-91.

79. American Heart Association. Part 2. Ethical Issues. *Circulation* 2005; 112:IV-6-IV-11.

80. Bailey ED, Wydro GC, Cone DC. Termination of resuscitation in the prehospital setting for adult patients suffering nontraumatic cardiac arrest. National Association of EMS Physicians Standards and Clinical Practice Committee. *Prehosp Emerg Care* 2000 April-June; 4(2):190-5.

Emergency Oxygen

When it is available, emergency oxygen can improve the care that you provide for any victim of a medical emergency. In this chapter you will learn the following:

- How important emergency oxygen is to emergency care
- The differences between oxygen for emergency care and for medical care

- The components of an emergency oxygen system
- How to assemble an emergency oxygen system
- How to handle emergency oxygen safely
- How to maintain an emergency oxygen system
- When and how to administer emergency oxygen

Importance of Emergency Oxygen

All sudden medical emergencies have the potential to cause oxygen to be depleted in the body. If left untreated, low oxygen levels (hypoxia) affect first the brain and then the heart and other organs. This can lead to respiratory arrest (breathing stops), cardiac arrest (heart stops), and eventually irreversible brain damage.

Health care providers and emergency responders such as EMTs routinely administer supplemental oxygen to ill or injured patients. Although it is believed that first aid use of emergency oxygen is helpful, there is no scientific evidence to prove it. In 2005, members of the National First Aid Science Advisory Board (NFASAB) examined the medical science literature to determine the feasibility and safety of recommending emergency oxygen in first aid.

They were unable to find any studies that evaluated the administration of emergency oxygen by first aid providers. As a result, their treatment recommendations state "There is insufficient evidence to recommend for or against the use of oxygen by the first aid provider.[8]"

Although scientific evidence for the use of emergency oxygen is lacking, health care providers and professional rescuers are nonetheless directed to give oxygen during basic and advanced life support as soon as it becomes available.[8] Laypersons have traditionally learned when and how to use emergency oxygen and rescue breathing devices in first aid courses sponsored by the American Red Cross, the American Safety & Health Institute, and other nationally recognized organizations. Given the

You must provide rescue breathing for victims who are not breathing.
Oxygen alone will not help!

potential benefit to the victim, it is reasonable for properly trained first aid providers to give emergency oxygen when it is available. This recommendation is based on common practices, although evidence-based guidelines recommend neither for or against its use.

The decision to have and use emergency oxygen should be based on its feasibility at a particular location or in a specific situation. If oxygen is available and you are trained to use it, include it as part of your first aid emergency care.

For the seriously ill or injured victim who is breathing normally, administering oxygen during an emergency increases the concentration of oxygen in the inhaled air. This increased oxygen concentration may prevent further deterioration of the victim's condition. For the victim who is not breathing, emergency oxygen fed into a barrier mask during CPR enriches the oxygen concentration of the breath being blown into

the victim by the rescuer. In either case, the amount of oxygen available to the victim is greatly increased.

Breathing in (inhalation) is active. The diaphragm and rib muscles contract to create a vacuum inside the chest, pulling air into the lungs. Breathing out (exhalation) is passive. The diaphragm and rib muscles return to a relaxed mode and air is then returned to the atmosphere.

When we inhale, we breathe approximately 21% oxygen from the atmosphere. Normally, we use about 5% of that oxygen in respiration. When we exhale, 16% (the unused portion of oxygen) leaves the lungs through the airway. This unused portion of oxygen can be used for rescue breathing. If emergency oxygen is added to your exhaled air during mouth-to-mask rescue breathing, the victim will receive at least 50% oxygen.

Oxygen in Emergency Care Versus Medical Care

Over the years there has been confusion about the legal regulations in the United States concerning the use of emergency oxygen and the need for a prescription. All oxygen cylinders are filled with what is known as "medical-grade" oxygen. The type of equipment that is attached to the cylinder and the intended use determine any restrictions or prescription requirements.

Oxygen equipment intended for emergency use (figure 5.1) can be purchased over the counter without a prescription (OTC), and anyone properly instructed in the use of emergency oxygen can administer it. Requirements for emergency use equipment are as follows:

- Emergency oxygen is in a portable cylinder with a regulator that provides oxygen for a minimum of 15 minutes.

- The device has a constant fixed-flow rate of not less than 6 liters per minute.

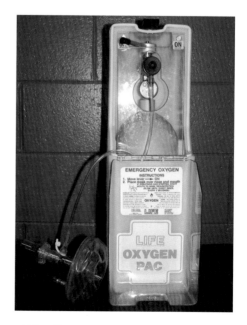

Figure 5.1   Emergency oxygen system.

- A content indicator gauge is present to determine how much oxygen is in the cylinder.

- The device is labeled "emergency" and has emergency operation instructions.

- A mask with a connection for oxygen tubing is supplied for oxygen administration.

If oxygen equipment is not intended for emergency use and is capable of providing less than 6 liters per minute, it requires a prescription.[1] The Food and Drug Administration requires a doctor's prescription for use of oxygen in medical applications, such as for persons with chronic lung disease or other conditions that require a varied flow and dosage of oxygen supply under the direction of a medical professional. The physician's staff or other personnel (e.g., EMS) may administer it as prescribed by the physician. Oxygen for medical use has a flow rate of 0 to 25 liters per minute that is controlled at the discretion of the operator. See figure 5.2.

In September 1996 the U.S. Food and Drug Administration (FDA), the regulatory agency for medical gases, determined that labeling for all oxygen equipment would bear the following statement: "WARNING: For emergency use only when administered by properly trained personnel for oxygen deficiency and resuscitation. For all other applications: CAUTION: Federal law prohibits dispensing without prescription."

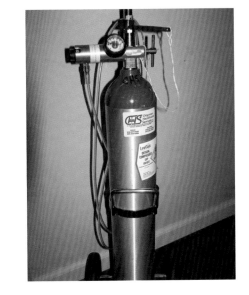

Figure 5.2   Medical oxygen system.

Even though the regulations at the federal level in the United States allow the use of emergency oxygen without a prescription, your local requirements may vary. Check the regulations that govern oxygen equipment or use in your location.

The training you receive as part of an emergency oxygen course is general in nature. To be considered properly trained to administer emergency oxygen, you must also have specific knowledge of the equipment you will use. You will need to become familiar with the manufacturer's directions and instructional materials provided with your system.

Components of an Oxygen System

An emergency oxygen system consists of these main components (figure 5.3):

- The *cylinder* holds the oxygen under pressure.

- The *regulator* controls how fast the oxygen flows from the cylinder.

- The *gauge* indicates how much oxygen is in the cylinder.

- The *tubing* carries the oxygen to the delivery point.

- The *delivery mask* is placed on the person's face so that oxygen can enter the person through the mouth and/or nose.

- The *case* safely secures the cylinder and other components.

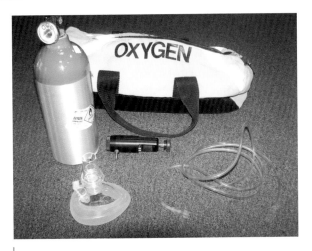

Figure 5.3   Components of an oxygen system.

Cylinder

The cylinder is constructed of steel or aluminum and is painted green for easy identification, and it comes in various sizes. Cylinder size is identified by a letter such as C, D, or E, and the size determines how much oxygen the cylinder can hold. Most emergency systems use a C-size cylinder, which provides about a 40-minute supply of oxygen.

A valve stem located on top of the cylinder is where the regulator is attached so that oxygen can safely flow out or where a filling device is attached to put oxygen back in. The valve stem has a special pin mount to prevent the cylinder from being filled with anything other than medical (USP)-grade oxygen. A washer is located at the connection point to help maintain a good seal; the washer is made of plastic, Teflon, nylon, or rubber with a metal ring.

The valve stem is used to turn the oxygen flow on and off. A handle may be built in, or a handle wrench may be needed. The handle wrench is supplied with the unit and should be securely attached with a chain.

When the oxygen supply runs out, most cylinders are refillable, although some are designed for one-time use and are disposable.

Regulator

A regulator is a device that attaches to the valve stem and decreases the content pressure to a safe delivery rate. Delivery rate is expressed in liters per minute (LPM or L/M). The regulator is tightened against the valve stem by turning a T-handle at the side of the regulator, and the oxygen flows out of the regulator through a tapered hose barb. You should know about and recognize the various types of regulators available so that you can select the one that is appropriate for your level of training.

Regulators come in three types:

- *Fixed flow* is the required regulator for use with emergency oxygen. Depending on the setting (6 or 12 LPM), such a system delivers a fixed flow of oxygen at a precise rate that cannot be adjusted. The oxygen constantly flows out at the fixed rate until it is turned off.

- *Variable flow* is the most common regulator used by medical professionals. It requires the user to set the amount of oxygen delivered from 0 to 25 LPM based on the patient's need, delivery device used, and protocol. The oxygen flows out constantly at the adjusted rate until it is turned off.

- *Demand regulators* deliver oxygen only when the person breathes in or, if fitted with a mechanical ventilator, when the provider pushes a button (similar to the function of a scuba regulator). This delivery system is highly efficient but requires specialized training and is for use by licensed medical professionals or specialized rescue personnel.

Gauge

The gauge (figure 5.4) indicates how much oxygen is available, but all gauges don't measure the same way. Become familiar with how the gauge on your system indicates the content level. The most common indicators are an empty-to-full scale, the pressure level inside the cylinder, or the time remaining in minutes.

If the gauge is built into the valve stem, it will read even when the flow is turned off. If the gauge is located on the regulator, the oxygen system must be turned on before the gauge will activate.

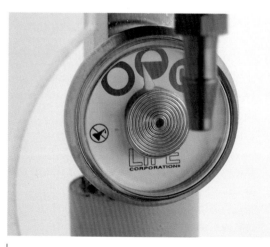

Figure 5.4   Gauge.

Tubing

The oxygen flows from the regulator to the delivery mask through crimp-proof plastic tubing. The tubing is attached to the regulator by slipping it over the hose barb, and it is attached to the delivery mask by slipping it over an oxygen inlet port.

Delivery Mask

Several types of oxygen delivery masks are available. You must know about and recognize the various types so that you can choose the delivery mask appropriate for your level of training and the condition of the victim.

Barrier Mask

The device most commonly used with emergency oxygen systems is a *barrier mask* with oxygen inlet and one-way valve (figure 5.5). The barrier mask is the same one that you use for CPR, but it is fitted with a port or inlet to which the oxygen tubing attaches. It is the ideal mask for delivering oxygen to either a breathing or nonbreathing victim. Sold under many brand names (Rescue Mask, Pocket Mask, SealEasy, to name a few), this mask is the one to consider for all emergency oxygen administration.

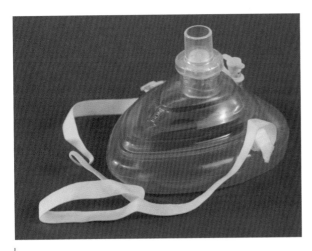

Figure 5.5   CPR mask.

Advantages

- It is easy to teach and learn its use.
- It can administer emergency oxygen to the breathing victim.
- It eliminates direct contact with the non-breathing victim's mouth or nose.
- It is easy to seal and deliver breaths to the nonbreathing victim, and it has been shown to provide the best ventilation when used by laypersons.[2]

Disadvantages

- The responsive victim may be apprehensive about the mask covering the face.
- The mask makes it slightly more difficult for the responsive victim to communicate verbally.
- Depending on the brand selected, the one-way valve may have to be removed to make it easier for the victim to breathe.

Nasal Cannula or Simple Face Mask

A *nasal cannula* or simple *face mask* is included with some emergency oxygen systems and is designed for use with victims who are breathing. A nasal cannula (figure 5.6) is a section of tubing that fits around the head and administers small quantities of oxygen directly into the nose. A simple face mask usually has an elastic strap that fits around the head and large ventilation holes in the mask that allow the oxygen flow to be diluted with air.

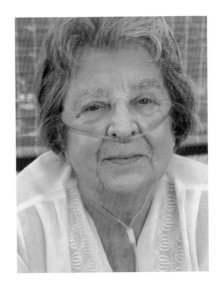

Figure 5.6   Nasal cannula.

Advantages

- The device can be held in place without assistance.
- It doesn't cause claustrophobia by covering the mouth and nose.
- It is nonthreatening.
- It is used for mild to moderate distress.

Disadvantages

- The concentration of oxygen is low.
- It can dry nasal membranes.
- It is less effective if the victim is breathing through the mouth.
- It can't be used for people who are not breathing.

Bag-Valve Mask

A *bag-valve mask* (figure 5.7) requires specialized training that is included in CPR courses for health care providers and professional rescuers. It is used only with nonbreathing victims to administer artificial ventilations. When connected to a supplemental oxygen source capable of delivering high-flow oxygen, the device stores oxygen in a bag that is filled from an oxygen reservoir. One rescuer holds the mask in place and another rescuer squeezes the bag to deliver the oxygen (see Skill Guides 1 and 4 on pages 118 and 123).

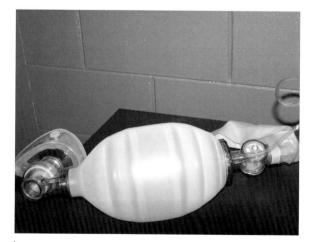

Figure 5.7 Bag-valve mask.

Advantages

- When connected to a high-flow (12 to 15 liters per minute) oxygen source, it delivers close to 100% oxygen.
- It eliminates the need for any mouth-to-mask contact.

Disadvantages

- It takes training and practice to master making a good seal and delivering oxygen efficiently without gastric distention (excess air in stomach). It may cause overinflation inconsistent with the 2005 guidelines.
- It usually requires at least two providers trained in its use.

Nonrebreather Mask

A nonrebreather mask requires specialized training and is to be used in a clinical setting by a licensed medical professional.

Advantage

It significantly increases the percentage of oxygen delivered.

Disadvantages

- It is not useful for someone who is not breathing.
- It may make the victim apprehensive about having the mask cover the face.
- It makes it more difficult to monitor the victim's airway and breathing.
- It makes it more difficult for the victim to talk.

Case

Keep your emergency oxygen system in a case to protect the components from damage and to provide easy access during an emergency. The most common types of cases are a wall-mounted hard case, a portable hard case, and a fabric bag with a carrying strap.

Assembly of Emergency Oxygen

Keep your oxygen system assembled and ready for immediate use. The only time you should take the system apart or assemble the components is for refilling, cleaning, or replacing parts. Follow these general steps when you want to remove the cylinder from an emergency oxygen system:

1. Turn the system off.
2. Loosen the regulator.
3. Lift the regulator off the valve stem.

Follow these steps when you assemble the components of an emergency oxygen system:[3]

1. Remove the protective seal on the cylinder valve stem (if present).
2. Connect the handle wrench, if the handle is not built in.
3. Quickly open and close the valve to test the flow and clean out any debris around the valve. Be sure the exit port (where the oxygen comes out) is directed away from you.
4. Check to make sure the sealing mechanism (gasket or washer) is in place on the regulator or at the connection to the tank stem.
5. Attach the regulator to the cylinder valve stem. Hand-tighten only.
6. Attach one end of the tubing to the hose nipple of the regulator.
7. Attach the other end of the tubing to the oxygen nipple or port of the mask.
8. Turn the system on and listen for oxygen flow.
9. Turn the system off and store for use.

Oxygen Safety

Emergency oxygen systems have three main safety concerns:

1. Oxygen inside the cylinder is compressed and highly pressurized.
2. Oxygen is chemically reactive and can interact with other chemical substances.
3. Oxygen supports combustion when a source of flame or spark is present.

Although oxygen cylinders are durable and safe under normal use, they are susceptible to damage from unprotected falls or inadvertent strikes. For example, if an oxygen cylinder should fall from a height and strike a hard surface, the valve head might break, causing rapid release of the contents (2,000 pounds per square inch [psi] or greater). The cylinder could "rocket," causing significant damage and personal injury or death depending on the contents' pressure.

Although oxygen is not flammable, it can react with other chemicals and create enough heat to initiate combustion or, in some cases, explosions. Oxygen also "feeds a fire," substantially increasing the rate at which flammable materials burn.

The Occupational Safety & Health Administration (OSHA), Compressed Gas Association (CGA), and other regulatory agencies have the same specific regulations for safe handling, use, and disposal of **all** compressed gas cylinders. Carefully read the Material Safety Data Sheet (MSDS) that accompanies the product.

The FDA has received more than a dozen reports in which regulators used with oxygen cylinders have burned or exploded, in some cases injuring personnel. The FDA and the National Institute for Occupational Safety and Health (NIOSH) believe that improper use of plastic gaskets or washers was a major factor in both the ignition and severity of the fires. The FDA and NIOSH recommend that the plastic crush gaskets commonly used to create the seal at the cylinder valve or regulator interface **never** be reused.[4] Reuse can deform the plastic gasket, increasing the likelihood that oxygen will leak around the seal and ignite. Also take the following general safety precautions:

- Always "crack" cylinder valves (open the valve just enough to allow gas to escape for a very short time) before attaching regulators in order to expel foreign matter from the outlet port of the valve.

- Always follow the regulator manufacturer's instructions for attaching the regulator to an oxygen cylinder.

- Always use the sealing gasket specified by the regulator manufacturer.

- Always inspect the regulator and seal before attaching it to the valve to ensure that the regulator is equipped with only one clean, sealing-type washer (reusable metal-bound rubber seal) or a **new** crush-type gasket (single use, not reusable, typically nylon) that is in good condition.

- Always be certain the valve, regulator, and gasket are free from oil or grease. Oil or grease contamination can contribute to ignition in oxygen systems.

- Tighten the T-handle firmly by hand, but do not use wrenches or other hand tools that may overtorque the handle.

- Open the post valve slowly. If gas escapes at the juncture of the regulator and the valve, quickly close the valve. Verify the regulator is properly attached and the gasket is properly placed and in good condition. If you have any questions or concerns, contact your supplier.

Reports have been made of patients and their bedding being set on fire during defibrillation when oxygen was in use. The oxygen concentration necessary to produce ignition will typically extend less than a foot in any direction from the oxygen source and will quickly disperse when removed. Therefore, you should remove the mask, place it several feet from the victim, and shut off the oxygen flow when delivering shocks. Leaving a device that continues to discharge oxygen near the victim's head before defibrillation is dangerous.

Other Safety Guidelines

Read and follow the specific maintenance, safety, and operating instructions provided with your system. These warnings apply to all oxygen systems:

- Never use oil, grease, adhesive tape, or other petroleum products on or near an oxygen cylinder or its components. A violent reaction can occur.

- Never smoke or use a match or lighter near oxygen systems.

- Turn off the oxygen flow and remove the oxygen system when delivering a shock with an AED.

- Emergency oxygen systems are not designed to be used in rescue situations as an air supply to the rescuer.

- Do not use emergency oxygen systems in oxygen-deficient atmospheres as a respirator or an air supply.

- Do not use emergency oxygen systems in a fire situation. Remove the victim from such dangers before using oxygen.

- Do not use emergency oxygen systems in hazardous or explosive environments. Remove the victim from such dangers before using oxygen.

Safe Storage Requirements

Here are some guidelines for storage of emergency oxygen:[5]

- Do not place containers where they might become part of an electrical circuit or arc.

- Do not expose compressed gas cylinders to extreme temperatures (more than 125 °F, or 51.6 °C).

- Keep valve protection caps on cylinders at all times except when cylinders are secured and connected to dispensing equipment.

- Do not store containers near readily ignitable substances or expose them to corrosive chemicals or fumes.

- Do not store containers near elevators, walkways, building entrances or exits, or unprotected platform edges or in locations where heavy moving objects may strike or fall on them.

- Secure all compressed gas cylinders in service or in storage at user locations to prevent them from falling, tipping, or rolling. Store and use them valve end up.

- Secure compressed gas cylinders with straps or chains connected to a wall bracket or other fixed surface or on a cylinder stand.

All compressed gases **must** be stored in areas away from heat, spark, flame sources, and explosive environments. If your facility maintains an extra supply of emergency oxygen cylinders, store them in a manner consistent with the guidelines described previously. Label the areas for **full** and **empty** cylinders.

Maintenance of Emergency Oxygen

Emergency oxygen systems are relatively maintenance free, but they need to be inspected on a regular basis to ensure the systems are ready for emergencies. After use during an emergency, the cylinder will need to be refilled (unless it is a disposable cylinder) and the components will need to be properly cleaned.

Inspections

Make inspection of your emergency oxygen system a regular part of your safety routine. Document your findings in a log. Conduct a visual inspection at least monthly that includes the following:

- See that no damage is visible to cylinders, regulators, or other components. Report damage to your safety or department manager immediately.

- Examine the content indicator gauge. Report cylinders that have not been used but that read "low" on the content indicator gauge as possibly having a leak. This helps ensure that there is adequate supply on hand when needed.

- Make sure the mask is present and that the one-way valve is attached and secure.

- Check that the tubing is not crimped and is securely attached to the hose barb on the regulator and the oxygen inlet on the mask.

- Ensure that any necessary handles or pins are present and attached by a chain.

- Make sure the components are clean and dry.

- Check the stability of the unit mount, rack, or holders.

Conduct an operational inspection when you first obtain your emergency oxygen system and after reassembly or at least every 6 months. Be sure to

1. turn the system on,
2. confirm oxygen flow, and
3. turn the system off and store it for use.

Refilling and Testing

When the gauge on your emergency oxygen system indicates less than half full, it's time to get the cylinder refilled. Any medical or industrial gas distributor that uses the Compressed Gas Association (CGA) #870 pin-indexed universal coupling for oxygen can refill cylinders. Look for these distributors in your phone directory under *welding equipment* and *gases.* Another option for refilling is to contact your local fire department or hospital and ask if they offer refill service for emergency oxygen systems.

Federal regulations in the United States and most countries require that an oxygen cylinder be visually inspected (internally and externally) and pressure tested every 5 years or at any time the cylinder shows evidence of dents, corrosion, cracked or abraded areas, leakage, thermal damage, or any other condition that might render it unsafe for use.[6] After a successful pressure test and inspection, a date is stamped into the cylinder. A cylinder is checked for a valid test date before it can be refilled. Federal regulations also require those who perform these cylinder tests to be currently approved to do so.[7] Disposable cylinders do not have this requirement, but they **must not** be refilled under any circumstances.

Cleaning

When an emergency oxygen system is used to provide care, the components are considered contaminated and must be replaced or cleaned. Cleaning procedures should follow bloodborne pathogen exposure and decontamination guidelines.

OSHA, CFR Title 29, Section 1910.1030 (bloodborne pathogens standard) states that all workplaces where employees have "reasonably anticipated" exposure to blood or other potentially infectious materials must have a written plan to protect employees from exposure to these materials. As with any item contaminated with blood or other potentially infectious material, a reusable oxygen cylinder or oxygen delivery device (mask, tubing, cannula) or other component that is visibly contaminated must be handled by a trained person who is wearing proper personal protective equipment. The cylinder or component can be initially surface-cleaned using warm, soapy water. It must be cleaned and disinfected with at least a 1:100 bleach-and-water solution or a commercial solution approved for use against biohazards.

Dispose of blood-soaked disposable components as biohazardous waste or disinfect them as described previously and dispose of them as regular waste. The biohazard symbol is displayed in figure 5.8. EMS personnel have containers on their units to dispose of these items. Ask if they will dispose of any contaminated materials for you.

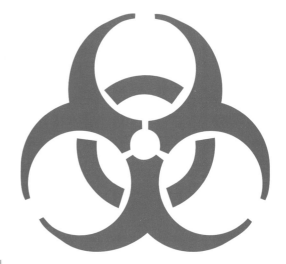

Figure 5.8   Biohazard symbol.

Have a policy in place for how you intend to dispose of these materials. If blood or any potentially infectious material is **not** present, disposable items are considered regular trash. If you are using emergency oxygen in your home, this regulation does not apply to you.

Now that you know how to operate an emergency oxygen system, review the following necessary steps in administering emergency oxygen to an injured or ill person.

Considerations in an Emergency Action Plan

You must answer at least four questions in order to be prepared to administer emergency oxygen:

1. How much oxygen should be kept on hand?

2. Where should the emergency oxygen unit be mounted or stored?

3. Who will bring emergency oxygen to the scene?

4. When will emergency oxygen be used?

Answer these questions **before** an emergency occurs, then practice your emergency action plan regularly. You don't want an emergency situation to be the first time you've put your plan to the test.

When you are deciding how much oxygen to keep on hand, a good rule is to determine the average EMS response time to your facility and have enough to last twice as long as the response time. In most circumstances, 30 minutes' to 1 hour's supply is sufficient. Also have an extra full cylinder to replace any that are off site being refilled or tested.

When you are deciding where the emergency oxygen unit should be mounted or stored, start with the storage guidelines listed previously in this chapter. Then identify a location that meets these guidelines and is easily accessible at all times. Do not store your emergency oxygen system in a locked closet. If it is necessary to lock up the system overnight, be sure that part of your daily opening procedure is to bring the system to a predetermined, accessible location.

When you are deciding who will bring the emergency oxygen to the scene, you must consider the number of people who will likely be present should an emergency occur. If you are the only trained person who will respond, you will either have to bring the emergency oxygen with you when you first recognize an emergency or ask bystanders to bring the emergency oxygen to the scene. If another trained person will usually be on site to respond, you must consider how an emergency situation will be communicated so that person will bring the emergency oxygen.

When you are deciding your protocol for when to use emergency oxygen, here are two good general rules to follow:

1. Use emergency oxygen any time serious signs and symptoms cause you to alert EMS (call 9-1-1).

2. Use emergency oxygen as soon as reasonably possible under the circumstances

Emergency oxygen can be used safely for any victim of a sudden illness or injury **unless** the victim is

- on fire;

- covered with grease, oil, or petroleum products;

- being shocked with an automated external defibrillator; or

- in a hazardous environment.

Administration of Emergency Oxygen

Integrate administering emergency oxygen into the emergency action steps you already know:

1. **Assess scene.** If the scene is not safe or at any time becomes unsafe, **get out!** Look for conditions that would make using emergency oxygen unsafe. Is there an open flame or a source of sparks? Are petroleum products or other chemicals present?

2. **Assess victim.** If there are serious signs and symptoms, follow steps 3 and 4:

3. **Alert EMS (call 9-1-1) or activate your emergency action plan.** Your plan should include alerting others to bring the emergency oxygen to the scene.

4. **Attend to the ABCDs.** Begin care based on the victim's symptoms. Add emergency oxygen when it arrives at the scene or as soon as reasonably possible.

The following instructions are a review of what you learned in the CPR chapter of this book. When you assess a victim, you look for serious signs and symptoms and the presence or absence of normal breathing:

- Breathing irregularly (too fast, too slow, too shallow, too deep)
- Wheezing, gurgling, or making high-pitched noises when breathing
- Feeling short of breath, dizzy, or light-headed
- Chest pain or tingling sensation in the extremities (arms, legs)
- Looking flushed, bluish, or pale

Alert EMS (call 9-1-1) if you see any of these signs and symptoms.

In the process of respiratory system failure, the brain will attempt to stimulate breathing. These *agonal* (close to death) attempts **do not** move enough air to sustain life. The victim will appear to be gasping, usually with the mouth opening during inspiration and closing during expiration, but little or no air movement will be present. Agonal respirations are slower and less frequent than normal respiratory effort. All too often, EMS personnel arrive at a scene and find would-be rescuers gathered around a victim with insufficient respirations; the rescuers "wait and see" if they should start rescue breathing or administer oxygen. If a victim is not breathing or appears not to be breathing enough (moving enough air) to support life, **you must alert EMS, begin CPR,** and preferably supplement your rescue breaths with emergency oxygen. Responding this way will not harm the person if he or she is breathing. However, do not simply put an oxygen mask on the victim and then "wait and see;" the victim may deteriorate to full cardiac and respiratory arrest.

If your assessment determines that a person is choking and the airway is obstructed by a foreign body, oxygen alone will not help. Follow the procedures for treatment of choking and obstructed airway for a conscious or unconscious person (as described in chapters 3 and 4). Administer emergency oxygen after the airway has been cleared.

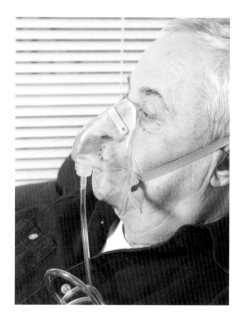

Do not assume that if the chest is moving an unresponsive person is breathing!
When in doubt, begin CPR.

Figure 5.9 shows the responses you should make for both breathing and nonbreathing victims.

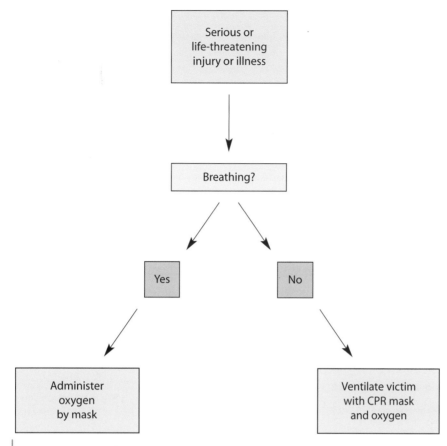

Figure 5.9 Deciding to administer oxygen.

Figure 5.10 shows the specific steps for helping a victim who is responsive and breathing, unresponsive and breathing, and unresponsive and not breathing normally.

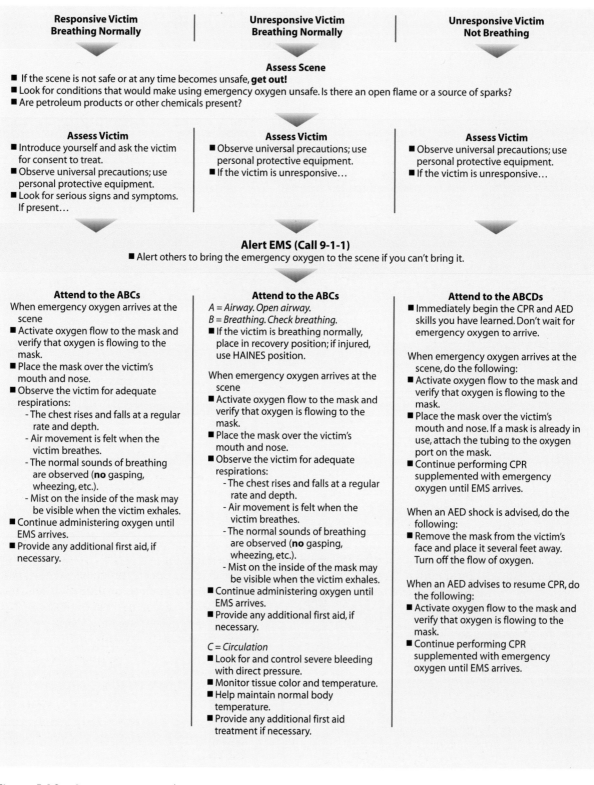

Responsive Victim Breathing Normally | **Unresponsive Victim Breathing Normally** | **Unresponsive Victim Not Breathing**

Assess Scene
- If the scene is not safe or at any time becomes unsafe, **get out!**
- Look for conditions that would make using emergency oxygen unsafe. Is there an open flame or a source of sparks?
- Are petroleum products or other chemicals present?

Assess Victim
- Introduce yourself and ask the victim for consent to treat.
- Observe universal precautions; use personal protective equipment.
- Look for serious signs and symptoms. If present…

Assess Victim
- Observe universal precautions; use personal protective equipment.
- If the victim is unresponsive…

Assess Victim
- Observe universal precautions; use personal protective equipment.
- If the victim is unresponsive…

Alert EMS (Call 9-1-1)
- Alert others to bring the emergency oxygen to the scene if you can't bring it.

Attend to the ABCs
When emergency oxygen arrives at the scene
- Activate oxygen flow to the mask and verify that oxygen is flowing to the mask.
- Place the mask over the victim's mouth and nose.
- Observe the victim for adequate respirations:
  - The chest rises and falls at a regular rate and depth.
  - Air movement is felt when the victim breathes.
  - The normal sounds of breathing are observed (**no** gasping, wheezing, etc.).
  - Mist on the inside of the mask may be visible when the victim exhales.
- Continue administering oxygen until EMS arrives.
- Provide any additional first aid, if necessary.

Attend to the ABCs
A = Airway. Open airway.
B = Breathing. Check breathing.
- If the victim is breathing normally, place in recovery position; if injured, use HAINES position.

When emergency oxygen arrives at the scene
- Activate oxygen flow to the mask and verify that oxygen is flowing to the mask.
- Place the mask over the victim's mouth and nose.
- Observe the victim for adequate respirations:
  - The chest rises and falls at a regular rate and depth.
  - Air movement is felt when the victim breathes.
  - The normal sounds of breathing are observed (**no** gasping, wheezing, etc.).
  - Mist on the inside of the mask may be visible when the victim exhales.
- Continue administering oxygen until EMS arrives.
- Provide any additional first aid, if necessary.

C = Circulation
- Look for and control severe bleeding with direct pressure.
- Monitor tissue color and temperature.
- Help maintain normal body temperature.
- Provide any additional first aid treatment if necessary.

Attend to the ABCDs
- Immediately begin the CPR and AED skills you have learned. Don't wait for emergency oxygen to arrive.

When emergency oxygen arrives at the scene, do the following:
- Activate oxygen flow to the mask and verify that oxygen is flowing to the mask.
- Place the mask over the victim's mouth and nose. If a mask is already in use, attach the tubing to the oxygen port on the mask.
- Continue performing CPR supplemented with emergency oxygen until EMS arrives.

When an AED shock is advised, do the following:
- Remove the mask from the victim's face and place it several feet away. Turn off the flow of oxygen.

When an AED advises to resume CPR, do the following:
- Activate oxygen flow to the mask and verify that oxygen is flowing to the mask.
- Continue performing CPR supplemented with emergency oxygen until EMS arrives.

Figure 5.10   Steps to oxygen administration.

If the mask seems too big for small children or infants, hold the mask close to their face and the oxygen will be drawn toward their face as they breathe. *If the mask seems too big for non-breathing small children or infants,* turn (rotate) the barrier mask upside down (nose area at the chin) if necessary (figure 5.11). This will allow you to make a seal and perform mouth-to-barrier mask rescue breathing.

If an adult victim cannot tolerate the mask on his or her face, hold the mask as close to the face as the victim will allow. The oxygen will be drawn toward his or her face as he or she breathes (figure 5.12). This will increase the amount of oxygen delivered to the victim.

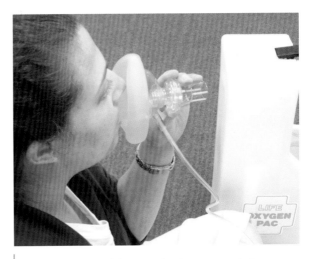

Figure 5.12 Holding mask above victim's face.

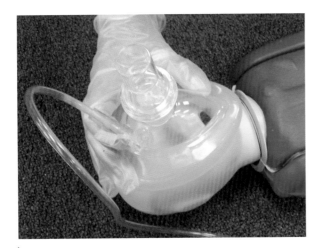

Figure 5.11 Rotating mask for child.

References

1. U.S. Food and Drug Administration. 2006. Review guidelines for oxygen generators and oxygen equipment intended for emergency use. www.fda.gov/cdrh/ode/doc986.pdf. Accessed 2006 August.

2. Paal P, et al. Comparison of mouth-to-mouth, mouth-to-mask and mouth-to-face-shield ventilation by lay persons. *Resuscitation* 2006 July; 70(1):117-23.

3. National Guidelines for First Aid Training in Occupational Settings. November 1998. Guidelines for a first aid oxygen administration enrichment program. www.ngfatos.net/downloads/ngfatos-o2.pdf. Accessed 2006 September.

4. U.S. Food and Drug Administration Center for Devices and Radiological Health and National Institute for Occupational Safety and Health. June 19, 2006. Public health notification: Oxygen regulator fires resulting from incorrect use of CGA 870 seals. www.fda.gov/cdrh/safety/042406-o2fires.html. Accessed 2006 August.

5. Compressed Gas Association. August 23, 2006. Safe handling of compressed gases in containers. http://www.cganet.com/publication_detail.asp?id=P-1. Accessed 2006 August.

6. U.S. Department of Transportation. Title 49—Transportation. October 1, 2002. Chapter I: Research and special programs administration. Part 180: Continuing qualification and maintenance of packagings. 49CFR180.205. http://hazmat.dot.gov/sp_app/approvals/regs/180.205-215.htm. Accessed 2006 August.

7. U.S. Department of Transportation Office of Hazardous Materials Safety. Pipeline and hazardous materials safety administration: Special permits and approvals to the hazardous materials regulations (HMR). http://hazmat.dot.gov/sp_app/approvals/exsys.htm. Accessed 2006 August.

8. American Heart Association and the American National Red Cross. Part 14: First aid oxygen. *Circulation* 2005;112:IV-197.

index

Note: The italicized *f* and *t* following pages numbers refer to figures and tables, respectively.

about the author

The **American Safety & Health Institute (ASHI)** is an association of approximately 35,000 professional safety and health educators and more than 5,500 training centers around the world. ASHI training center membership covers a wide range of organizations, including local emergency medical service, fire, rescue and law enforcement agencies, hospitals, universities, public school districts, community colleges, vocational schools, charitable foundations, local and federal governments, and public and private corporations and training companies. ASHI's mission is to continually improve safety and health education by promoting high standards for members, principles of sound research for curriculum development, and the professional development of safety and health instructors worldwide.